Farhad

# Tai Chi

## for fitness over forty

# Tai Chi

## for fitness over forty

### Relaxation exercises for good health

Grandmaster Gary Khor

Foreword by Dr Nigel Hope

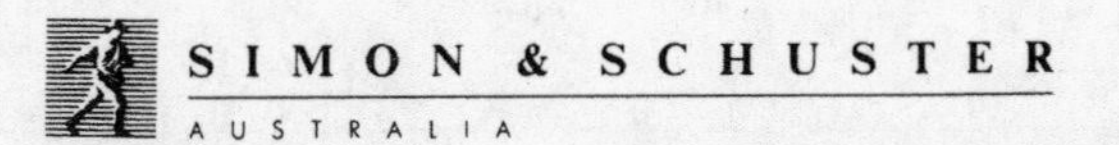

The advice given in this book is not intended as a substitute for advice from your medical practitioner. The program could be used effectively to promote general health and/or as an introduction to Tai Chi-based exercise. While all the exercises and techniques advised are generally safe, your medical practitioner knows your specific medical condition and you should discuss this program with him/her before you begin.

First published in Australia in 2002 by
Simon & Schuster (Australia) Pty Limited
20 Barcoo Street,
East Roseville NSW 2069

A Viacom Company
Sydney New York London

Visit our website at www.simonsaysaustralia.com



National Library of Australia
Cataloguing-in-Publication data:

Khor, Gary, 1947– .
Tai chi for fitness over forty : relaxation exercises
for good health.

Includes index.
ISBN 0 7318 1144 5.

1. T'ai chi ch'üan. 2. Relaxation. 3. Health. I. Title.

613.7148

Cover photograph: Getty Images
Cover and internal design: Greendot Design
Illustrator: Lorenzo Lucia
Typeset in Bembo 12pt on 14pt leading
Printed in Australia by Ligare Book Printer

10 9 8 7 6 5 4 3 2 1

# Contents

# Acknowledgments

THIS BOOK IS THE RESULT of 25 years of research from Tai Chi classes conducted throughout Australia. The Australian Academy of Tai Chi has over 200 instructors who constantly help update the research program. I would like to take this opportunity to thank each and every one of them for their assistance and contribution.

In particular I wish to thank David Walker for his research work and effort in helping to put this book together. My sincere appreciation to Dr Nigel Hope for his kind words and endorsement of our work. And finally, my thanks to the editors, designer, illustrator and the staff at Simon & Schuster (Australia).

GRANDMASTER GARY KHOR

# Foreword by Dr Nigel Hope

HOW IS IT THAT I AM WRITING a foreword for a book based on traditional Chinese healing techniques? As an orthopaedic surgeon specialising in knee surgery and sports medicine, I am well-versed in the scientific western technologies of arthroscopic surgery, ligament reconstruction and joint replacement. In addition, I undertook an extensive period of study of the structure, function, and repair capacity of the supportive (connective) tissues of the knee joint, culminating in a PhD in this field. Thus, my medical perspective is that of the pragmatic and traditional western 'clinician–scientist'.

One would think the fundamental axiom of causality dictated by my western training would leave no place for the oriental 'magic' of the Tai Chi system. However, I share a paradoxical experience with C. G. Jung, the noted academic–psychiatrist who found himself writing the foreword to Richard Wilhelm's translation of *I Ching*. Jung quite eloquently summed up the situation as '…[a foreword] from my hand must be a testimonial of my individual experience…'

I practised 'hard/external' martial arts forms for over 20 years and have been active in western-style sports and fitness training my entire life. The impact nature of most western sport forms and 'external' martial arts, such as Karate and Tae Kwon Do, tend to focus upon aerobic fitness and explosive manoeuvres. Ultimately, and more often than not, just as professional athletes are plagued by and prematurely terminated by injury so too the amateur sportsman suffers a similar fate as one's 40th birthday approaches. Gradually, I was forced by injury and physiology (aging) to re-evaluate the punishing forms of these types of training.

My wife, in her gentle and timely way, suggested I join her in Tai Chi practice. My initial resistance to the practice as being 'too soft' was immediately addressed as I struggled to complete a simple set of exercises under the instruction of a practitioner ten years older than myself. I considered myself to be 'fighting fit' at this time, so the resultant cognitive dissonance beckoned resolution. I also began to appreciate I was aiming for health far closer to life 'after 40' than 'before 40'.

My personal experience of Tai Chi began to alter my perceptions of exercise, fitness and health. I began to experience a different type of fitness. Instead of feeling exhausted as I had after a weight-lifting session, a long road run, or a sparring (fighting) session in the dojo, I felt energised and ready for more after a session of Tai Chi. My observations led me to conclude that western sport and exercise may not necessarily be synonymous with health, particularly considering the high injury rates.

I became more interested in forms of exercise that allowed me to exercise my body and also benefited my mind and spirit. Tai Chi is distinctive in its slow and graceful movements; it is based on a 'soft internal school' of Chinese martial art. It is also a form of 'moving meditation'. It is best summarised by Grandmaster Khor: '…underneath this veneer of carefree softness lies a complex art which draws its health theory from traditional Chinese medicine and its guiding principles from the Chinese philosophy of the *Tao* (the way of nature).'

I met Grandmaster Gary Khor through my practice and study of Khor-style Tai Chi. I was asked to become an official member of the Australian Academy of Tai Chi Medical Review Committee in 2001. I was happy to accept this opportunity to participate in a forum that ensures the programs and services provided by the AATC are soundly based on the health perspectives of both western and oriental medicine. Although I have no expertise in oriental medicine, I am able to bring to the Academy considerable expertise in western medicine.

The enduring health benefits of Khor-style Tai Chi provide a much needed alternative for the ageing athlete. This experience challenged my personal philosophy of 'no pain, no gain', which seems to pervade Western thought. It initiated extensive research into the subject, which culminated in my personal commitment to Tai Chi practice. The multiple benefits of this form are well-documented in Grandmaster Khor's books. The painless acquisition of health is there for the taking. This is the basis of the oriental philosophy, which has my experiential support.

Osteoarthritis is something everyone experiences if they live long enough. This progressive condition eventually destroys the bearing surfaces of joints and necessitates their complete replacement, usually in older patients but not exclusively. This type of salvage surgery is extremely effective in reducing pain, increasing motion, and improving overall joint function; however, it involves a major surgical procedure, extensive removal of biological tissue and replacement with synthetic components (metal/plastic) that require changing every ten years. Less destructive partial joint replacements are now being implanted, but the biological alternatives of cartilage transplantation fails in one third of cases. Hopefully, the new technology of tissue engineering may make possible the replacement of damaged tissue with part-synthetic and part-biological materials.

Western medicine's knowledge of osteoarthritis as a disease process was dramatically altered in the early 1980s with the advent of the minimally invasive (keyhole) technique that allowed early examination of arthritic joints. However, as is the paradigm of Western medicine, it is the effects of arthritic disease that have been extensively examined while prevention strategies are rarely discussed. This is where it may be prudent to examine oriental medicine and philosophical thought.

The Tai Chi system has been developed and successfully practiced for over a millennium. It is only in relatively recent times that this ancient system has become available in the West. The appeal of the Tai Chi for Fitness Over Forty (FOF) program is that it does not require years of dedicated Tai Chi training to be of benefit. Grandmaster Khor has extracted the healing techniques from multiple Tai Chi forms. These techniques are the essence of the forms.

Tai Chi FOF program focuses on performing these exercises rather than practicing the extended Tai Chi form. Thus, it provides an easier and targeted introduction to the beneficial aspects of Tai Chi. This book also provides a well-written and easy-to-understand description of body–mind medicine. The FOF system is elegantly revealed. A detailed review of the manuscript indicates a solid, Western scientific foundation integrated with the ancient, experiential wisdom of the East.

Here is the distilled essence of Tai Chi. Practised mindfully it will heal and enhance your quality of life after 40! It is with great pleasure that I commend to you this book.

DR NIGEL HOPE
MB, BS (Syd), PhD (Syd), FRACS, FAOrthA
Honorary Associate, Faculty of Medicine, University of Sydney

# PART 1

# Living Longer, Living Better

# Life After Age 40 in the Third Millennium

YOU'VE PROBABLY HEARD the saying 'life begins at 40' but perhaps your experience might be more that 'life begins to show at 40'!

Certainly, as you approach or pass this age, it is likely that you will become more and more aware of health issues and how they can impact on the quality of life you want to lead. For instance, if you have played vigorous and active sports, you may be noticing an increasing frequency of injury and the fact that it takes longer to recover from such injury. On the other hand, if you have led a largely sedentary life, you may be beginning to notice other problems, such as a reduction in stamina, energy and flexibility.

Even if you have not yet experienced any of these things, you are almost certainly beginning to notice a rising incidence of medical 'issues' among your friends and acquaintances of this age group. The condition and health of surviving parents may also cause you to reflect on what you might expect from life as you move into its later stages.

Most people born in the latter half of the 20th century are starting to become aware that, unlike generations born in previous centuries (who considered themselves lucky to survive a few years beyond the end of their working lives), they face the prospect of a reasonable percentage of their lives being spent in the 'post retirement' period. These days at age 40 you can expect, on average, to have as many years ahead of you as behind you. Whether we find this prospect encouraging or discouraging reflects on what we feel will be the quality of this period of life.

What implications are there then for this extended post-retirement period? Well, for one thing, health experts are now starting to talk of the 'Third' and 'Fourth' stages of life rather than 'old age' or 'retirement'. These new terms are considered necessary to spell out a very important distinction in how we live our lives in these periods.

The Third Stage of life is seen as a positive and enjoyable period of life that takes place after you have finished your formal working life (or finished raising your family). You are still living an active and independent life and you may well be making significant social contributions or perhaps exploring and developing skills, hobbies and travel that you did not have time for during your working life.

The Fourth Stage is that negative period of your life when deteriorating health has made you dependent on others for care and attention. You no longer live an independent life and this period is regarded as being of low quality. Obviously, you want to live a life where you spend a long a time in the Third Stage and little or no time in the Fourth.

If you keep yourself healthy then the Third Stage of your life may well amount to a period of 20 or 30 years. If, on the other hand, you fail to maintain your health then, with the medical technology now available, the dependent, low-quality Fourth Stage of life may grow to cover that 20–30 year period! This is unlikely to be something that you cheerfully contemplate! In fact, the prospect is so depressing that many people choose not to think about the Fourth Stage and the life ahead of them. Consequently, they fail to take a few simple steps that can prolong the Third Stage and vastly improve their prospects of having a long, healthy and enjoyable life.

## Understanding the ageing process

The first thing that we have to understand is that feebleness of mind and body are not natural consequences of ageing, but more a result of the lifestyle that we adopt as we age. Nature seems to have one inviolable rule: 'Use it or lose it!' If we do not exercise the mind, body and emotions then these functions degrade.

We have all met older people who are more alert and active than much younger people. When we meet such a person, we should not regard them as a miraculous occurrence. This is what we should all expect as we advance through our lives. Too often we have a blinkered view and believe that such people are lucky to be healthy and alert, able to walk for miles, maintain interests in hobbies and creative pursuits, and assist in the community. We should realise that the very health and alertness of these older people comes from engaging in these activities, not the other way around!

It is said that, in 2800 BC, the Emperor Huang Di looked at the landscape around his capital after a flood from the Yellow River and saw the water became stagnant and polluted as it lay still. Not only did it look and smell bad, but disease was rampant. Since Huang Di believed that mankind was simply a reflection of nature, he had no difficulty in drawing the conclusion that, if human beings became still and sedentary, they would also stagnate, their minds and bodies would deteriorate, and illness and disease would follow. So the Emperor decreed that his subjects should perform specially designed 'health dances' to maintain their fitness and prevent disease. This was perhaps the first 'Life Be In It' campaign—some 4800 years ago!

Millennia later, our scientific studies are showing that the things we tend to associate with old age, such as loss of muscle tone, need not occur if we maintain an active lifestyle, and that IQ relates not so much to age as to the mental activities that we perform. The studies are also finding that the more we engage with others, even pet animals, the fitter we are becoming and the longer we are living.

This does not mean that there are not physical changes that occur as we age. The speed of cellular regeneration is slower, and so it takes longer to repair damage to the body. Our digestive systems do not work as efficiently and our immune systems are not as effective. Our hearing and sight also tend to deteriorate, although there are many people of advanced years who have good sight and hearing.

To have a long and healthy life, firstly, we need to know what we can do with our lifestyles to offset or even prevent these physical changes—for example, how we exercise, how we eat, what stresses we put ourselves under, and what type of environment we create around us.

Another aspect of lifestyle-related ageing is that the body can start to 'rust'. Just as a piece of iron oxidises (or reacts with the oxygen to break down into iron oxide) so, too, the body can start to oxidise as cells and tissues are broken down. This is the work of the notorious free radicals.

Essentially, free radicals are simply positive ions. (Most of the body's chemicals have a negative charge.) The free radicals come along and bond with the negative charge of the body's atoms, effectively interfering with the atom's function and the structure it forms. If this happens frequently enough, then the whole structure collapses.

The 'rusting' of the body is largely due to the presence of these free radicals in our environment. Unfortunately, the society that we have created is a highly toxic one, loaded with these destructive positive ions. Again, however, this process is not inevitable.

Have you ever noticed how some new cars become rusted-out wrecks within the space of a few years, while other older cars remain shining and gleaming decades later. The difference is the care that has been taken with them—the 'health care' that they have been given. Likewise, if we want to slow down the 'rusting' of our bodies, we can begin by doing the following:

- reducing the toxic load in our living environment;
- ensuring our diets contain lots of antioxidants to combat these positive ions; and
- making sure our circulatory systems operate efficiently, so that the antioxidants are effectively delivered to all parts of the body.

In addition to the damage caused by positive ions, our bodies take longer to repair as we age. However, we can offset this problem by:

- reducing the amount of damage that our body has to repair in the first place (this can be achieved by the same actions as mentioned above);
- reducing 'stress', because stress has a damaging effect on many of the body's systems; and
- making sure that the body has all the dietary resources that it needs to maintain itself (such as minerals, vitamins, proteins and carbohydrates).

## The Fitness Over Forty (FOF) Program

Many people seem to regard health as being the absence of sickness, but the aims of the Fitness Over Forty (FOF) Program go far beyond creating this condition. The FOF Program aims to create a state where we feel vital and full of energy. Mentally, we are alert, positive and optimistic. Physically, our bodies have stamina, good muscle tone, suppleness and flexibility. Both mentally and physically, we feel balanced and coordinated.

> AIMING FOR HEALTH, ENERGY, VITALITY AND WELL-BEING.

This approach can have real consequences. Focusing on positive aspects of life has a much more beneficial effect than focusing on negative aspects. Getting up every morning and saying 'I am not sick' is not as beneficial as getting up and saying 'I am healthy!' The reason for this is that your subconscious works with images rather than words. Summoning up the image of sickness rather than health simply programs the subconscious with continual images of sickness.

For instance, if you have a health issue, such as arthritis, the focus should not be on controlling the arthritic condition and reducing pain but on becoming supple and flexible with free and easy joint movement. The focus needs to be shifted from being a focus on disease to a focus on health. We are not aiming to avoid arthritis or reduce the pain of arthritis, we are aiming to feel full of energy and vitality.

## Preparing for health throughout life

The fact that you have read this far indicates that not only do you want a high quality Third Stage of life (we all want that), but that you are also prepared to make an effort to at least find out how to achieve this objective. In this you have taken an important step. You have started your journey. Now, you need a vehicle that will allow you to travel quickly and safely to your destination.

In short, you need to establish a 'health maintenance program'—a series of exercises and approaches to life that will not only keep your mind and body in a healthy condition but, in so far as it is possible, repair any pre-existing damage and minimise the 'quality of life impacts' of any condition that you might have developed or be developing.

There are a number of questions that you might have about a health maintenance program, such as:

- Why start a health maintenance program?
- How does the FOF Program work?

- Is the FOF Program affordable?
- Will the FOF Program come with a 'misery factor'? That is, will it involve transferring the potential misery and boredom from later parts of life into earlier parts through bland diets, hours of repetitious and mind-numbing exercises, and a general forgoing of the 'pleasures of life'?

## WHY START A HEALTH MAINTENANCE PROGRAM?

To convince ourselves we need to start a health maintenance program, we need to find health approaches that generate a high-quality old age. In my travels around China I was continuously impressed by the fact that some of the best Tai Chi and Qigong I had ever seen was performed by masters who were 70, 80 and even 90 years old!

In most sports and physical pursuits, practitioners are well past their peak at the grand old age of 40! However, these masters seemed to have a special magic in their movements. They moved with rhythm, grace and coordination. They were flexible, well balanced, mentally alert, and full of vital energy. When I watched them, I knew that this is how I wanted to be at their age. Not stiff, arthritic, short of breath and energy, mentally dull, and suffering a host of complaints and ailments. There was obviously something about their lifestyle and approach to life that had resulted in this high quality of life. Was it something that could be transferred to our modern lifestyle, or were these last relics of a traditional Chinese approach to life impracticable in our world of today?

When the communists took control of China, they regarded Tai Chi as elitist (and somewhat dangerous in terms of its philosophical approach to life), and so it was thought that the 'old' or 'traditional' cultural relics, such as Tai Chi and Qigong, would not last long in the 'New China'. However, those who form the communist government of China had always been great pragmatists and they had a major problem. The medical infrastructure they had inherited from the previous nationalist government was in shambles. It would be years, decades, before it could be built into an effective system. How could the pressure be taken off the medical system until it had been properly reconstructed?

The answer was relatively simple. Keep people healthy and they would not need to use the medical system as much.

After much investigation, it was found that Tai Chi and other Qigong arts were the best way of keeping the population healthy and so minimise demands on the medical infrastructure. As soon as this was known, massive public education systems encouraging the use of Tai Chi and Qigong were put into place. Hence we have seen photographs of hundreds, even thousands, of Chinese citizens performing Tai Chi in such places as 'the Bund' in Shanghai.

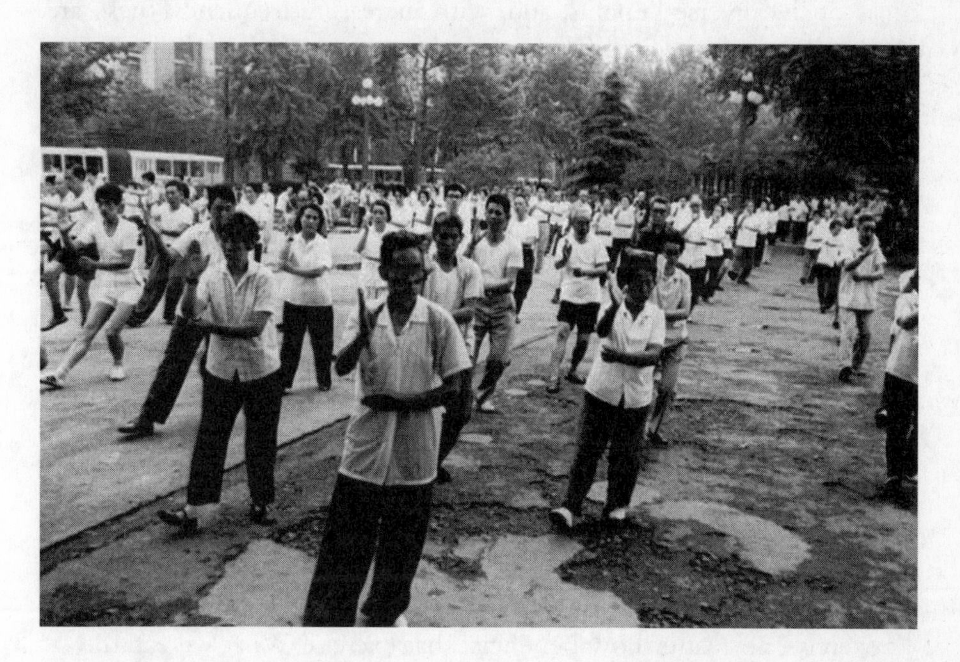

In many ways, this marked a renaissance in traditional Chinese health approaches. Not only was the new Chinese state sufficiently impressed with the results to continue and strengthen their programs but 'traditional' arts such as Tai Chi and Qigong, not to mention acupressure and herbs, have also aroused significant interest throughout the world.

So, is the problem already solved? Do we simply have to teach everyone to practice Tai Chi and Qigong to solve all their health problems as they age? If only it were so simple!

In 1976, when I began teaching Tai Chi in Australia, most people thought that Tai Chi was an item you ordered at a Chinese restaurant! Even after developing simpler techniques for teaching and learning Tai Chi, after 25 years the Academy has taught only slightly more than 100,000 Australians. At the same time, other Australian Tai Chi instructors may have reached another 50,000 or so students. In all, 150,000 people out of 12 million or so is scarcely one per cent of the country's adult population. The penetration of Tai Chi and Qigong into other countries tends to be even lower! We are going to have to do much better than this if we are going to use these arts to make serious improvements in overall health and quality of the life.

What are the reasons why more people do not take up Tai Chi or Qigong? Certainly, there is no problem with credibility. Most people know of the diverse benefits, and, with increasing frequency, these are being confirmed by scientific research. Also, many medical practitioners who recognise the benefits are referring their patients to Tai Chi. So why aren't more people doing it? The reasons include:

- Many people do not want to spend years learning and refining the Tai Chi form, particularly in terms of its martial arts aspects. On the other hand, the 'instant Tai Chi' approach is rightly suspect as being near to useless.
- In some senses, the 'holistic' nature of Tai Chi works against it—while Tai Chi raises the overall health of the body (allowing the body to better maintain its overall functioning and resolve many existing problems), today's generation is brought up to be focused on 'symptoms' or problems. If a person has, or is concerned about, a health issue (such as a circulatory problem, osteoporosis, depression or lack of balance), then they want to be working directly on that problem.
- People also recognise that there is more to a healthy life than exercise, no matter how beneficial that exercise. What we eat, the environment that we live in, and the 'style' of life that we lead all impact on our health.

### HOW DOES THE FOF PROGRAM WORK?

The FOF Program is designed to resolve the issues listed above. It uses simple and easy-to-learn exercises, but it is not an 'instant Tai Chi' or 'instant Qigong' approach. The FOF Program exercises incorporate the essential elements and principles of traditional Chinese approaches to health with the latest knowledge and understanding of the functioning of the mind and body.

You won't have to spend a large amount of time exercising, but it is certainly more than the 'two-minutes-a-day' approach. (The reasons why we need to exercise for more than 20 minutes at a time are discussed later.) And, importantly, the FOF Program exercises are invigorating rather than exhausting, stimulating rather than demanding.

The FOF Program is constructed of four health modules. These are Exercise, Breathing and Meditation, Acumassage and *Chi* Nutrition/

Environment. Each of these is dealt with individually, and each works in its own right. However, by using all of the modules together, you will achieve more easily a healthy life, from beginning to end.

### IS THE FOF PROGRAM AFFORDABLE?

Good news! The FOF Program is designed around the use of your mind and body. This is all you will need for the Exercise, Breathing and Meditation, and Acumassage modules. You can also implement most of the benefits in the Nutrition/Environment module at very low cost, although if you choose to use certain supplements to prevent or control specific conditions then the cost might increase slightly.

You do not need any special clothes or equipment, and you can practice in your home or back garden. The FOF Program is a health approach that you can take anywhere.

### WILL THE FOF PROGRAM COME WITH A 'MISERY FACTOR'?

It often seems that to avoid the possibility of unpleasant things in the future, we have to do unpleasant things in the now. This can be a powerful disincentive to taking immediate action. Who knows? We might just get away with it!

Fortunately, with the FOF Program, you do not need to take this gamble. There is no transfer of misery from one part of your life to another. You will find is that the exercises are both interesting and enjoyable to perform. Your diet can remain pleasant and stimulating. And, the program not only pays off years later, it pays off immediately—with improved vitality and well-being, better coordination and balance, improved muscle tone, and a more effective immune system.

## Who is the FOF Program for?

While you are never too old to start the FOF Program, you are never too young either! Just as we use our childhood to prepare ourselves for the adult phase of our lives, the sooner we begin preparing our body and mind for the Third Stage of life the better the results will be.

I am also a great believer in the fact that we live in the 'now' not the future and that the 'now' should never be sacrificed to the future. Therefore, the FOF Program, while aiming to improve your future is also designed as a fun and interesting program to be enjoyed now. The FOF Program is suitable for anyone in reasonable health, however, if you have a specific health problem, always consult your doctor before undertaking any health exercise program or dietary change. If you have an existing health issue, the FOF Program is designed to work in conjunction with other treatments provided by health professionals—it does not replace those treatments for your condition. And, while following the FOF Program can improve a health issue by improving your total well-being, you should never alter medication or treatment for a specific condition without discussing this with your doctor.

With regard to children, the FOF Program is beneficial but do remember that it is designed for more mature people. Children need to have a program that is specifically tailored to their attention span and interests as well as their health and well-being.

PREVENTION IS BETTER THAN CURE.

**THE FOF PROGRAM AND HEALTH OVER 40**

The FOF Program has benefits for most of the health conditions that are associated with people aged over 40 because it works on a holistic level. The program recognises that the healthier each body function is, the better the body can deal with specific health issues that may arise. On the other hand, symptom-based approaches that focus on specific problems can ignore, or even damage, other body systems. For example, exercising to improve the health of your heart has little benefit if you are also causing deterioration of the muscular system; this is because the tone and health of the muscles directly relate to the amount of stress put on the heart.

So, while the selection of exercises and techniques that form the FOF Program are designed to assist with specific health areas associated with ageing, they also benefit many conditions and not just those which are listed here. Some of the more common conditions of 'modern' ageing, and addressed in the FOF Program, are:

- cancer and immune-deficiency problems;
- arthritis;
- osteoporosis;
- circulatory problems and loss of muscle tone and flexibility;
- deteriorating digestive function;

- reduction in coordination and balance, and increased exposure to falls;
- fatigue, depression and loss of vitality.

Note that asthma is not included in the above listing because, while the condition is very important, it is not, strictly speaking, an ageing disease (and is, in fact, much more prevalent in children).

### LIFE AFTER THE FOF PROGRAM

If you have just started the program, probably the last thing you're concerned about is what you're going to do after you have your FOF Program up and running. Indeed, if the FOF Program is so good, why should you need to do anything else?

From a health viewpoint, you do not have to move on from this program. However, most people are always seeking new challenges and they do not want to do the same thing, year in and year out. Therefore, the FOF Program takes great care to ensure that it can grow as you grow.

You do not have to give it away to try something else—the FOF Program can remain as the core of an overall health program that can grow in many directions. Personally, I also hope that participants in the program will find the exercises and techniques so enjoyable and beneficial that they will become interested in expanding their knowledge about the areas from which these were drawn. For instance:

- The FOF Exercise module may encourage you to learn a Tai Chi or a Qigong form such as the Wild Goose, the Lohan, or the Shibashi. There are many appropriate forms to consider, and they can benefit particular health issues, age groups or lifestyles.
- The techniques in the FOF Breathing and Meditation module can be supplemented with other *Chi* meditation forms and deeper work on the Microcosmic Orbit.
- The techniques provided in the FOF Acumassage module can be built upon to include forms, such as Dragon *Chi* massage, which can be used in everyday life.
- The FOF *Chi* Nutrition/Environment module focuses on diet—how you buy, store, prepare, mix, cook and present food is a whole fascinating study in itself—and the environmental issues which can be combined with the Chinese art of Feng Shui (an art that aims to provide a healthy energetic environment).

### THE FOF PROGRAM AND TAI CHI

While the practice of Tai Chi forms and practice of the FOF Program work well on their own, there are advantages in combining the two disciplines. For instance, if you already know and practice Tai Chi, the FOF Program can be a great supplement that increases your understanding of Tai Chi and the benefits that you can obtain from it. If you do not know Tai Chi, but would like to learn, the FOF Program is a great starting point. By becoming familiar with the FOF exercises, it will be easier to begin to learn Tai Chi.

Note that if you do intend to learn Tai Chi, you should choose a qualified instructor.

## How to use the FOF Program modules

In the following parts of the book, you will find the exercises and techniques that make up the modules of the FOF Program. They are:

- Exercise module;
- Breathing and Meditation module;
- Acumassage module; and
- *Chi* Nutrition/Environment module.

While the best results are obtained by using all the modules of the program together, following just one is better than using none of them at all. You may also choose to gradually introduce the program with one or more modules at a time.

To further enhance your knowledge and practice of the modules of the FOF Program, five appendices have been provided covering:

- the benefits of and techniques for healthy relaxation;
- how to achieve a healthy posture;
- healthy movement techniques;
- healthy breathing techniques; and
- the energy system that comprises the meridians and acupoints.

Throughout the book there may be a number terms you may not be familiar with. Please refer to the glossary at the back of the book. There is also a section advising of classes and other resources for further study.

We hope you enjoy and benefit from the FOF Program.

Part 2

# The FOF Program Exercise Module

# The Exercise Module

AS INDICATED BY ITS NAME, this module deals with the physical exercise element of the program. While practice of this module will increase your stamina, develop musculature and consume calories, these are not the main objectives of the module. Rather the exercises in this module are designed to maintain and enhance the body's health at a holistic level.

## The FOF Exercise module sets

The exercise sets included in the FOF Exercise module are:

- Set 1 Quiet Standing exercises
- Set 2 Neck and shoulder exercises
- Set 3 Waist exercises
- Set 4 Finger, elbow and wrist exercises
- Set 5 Toe, ankle, knee and hip exercises

### HOW MANY OF THE EXERCISES SHOULD YOU DO?

There may be reasons why performance of one or more of the exercises is not possible or appropriate for you but, generally speaking, you should strive to do as many of the exercises as possible in each set of the module. This does not mean that you have to do all the exercises of every set at one time. For example, you may choose to spread the exercises over a three-day period.

### HOW LONG SHOULD EACH EXERCISE PERIOD BE?

Unless there are medical reasons to the contrary, you should strive to exercise for continuous periods of 20 minutes or more. The initiation of the relaxation response, and its maintenance for a period of at least 20 minutes, is most important.

At a neurological or electrochemical level, many of us can learn to relax quite quickly—shifting the mind over to alpha-wave production in a matter of seconds. The body, however, is basically biochemical. It takes time for the body's levels of stress chemicals to be reduced, but, generally, this can be achieved if the mind remains relaxed for 20 minutes. If both the body and the mind are relaxed at the end of the session, then the period of time before we become stressed again will be extended. This is not just a matter of feeling good for longer. Our health is dependent on the ratio of time that we spend in the relaxation response compared to the stress response—the more relaxation in this ratio the better our health.

Studies have shown that when you take a group of people who have just performed a period of relaxing exercise and give them a stressful task to perform, the relaxing exercise that shows the slowest increase in stress levels is Tai Chi.

### HOW OFTEN SHOULD YOU EXERCISE EACH WEEK?

Again, unless there are medical reasons to the contrary, plan to spend at least 2 hours per week exercising (with a period of at least 40 minutes every three days). For each exercise in this module, the suggested length of time or number of repetitions is provided as a minimum guideline.

At least three of these exercise sessions per week are necessary if you are going to see any significant improvements in your health, but do not go to the opposite extreme. Many of us get very enthusiastic about things when we first start off but more exercise does not necessarily mean more health benefits. An old Tai Chi story explains the fallacy:

> A keen student once approached his Tai Chi Master to ask how long it would be before he would succeed in mastering his Tai Chi. The Master asked to watch the student's Tai Chi and then questioned him about his

training program. After some deliberation, the Master advised the student it would take him about two years more to master that form. The student was clearly disappointed about the length of time. So he asked the Master how long it would take if he doubled the amount of training he did. The Master answered that this was a difficult question, but it would probably take the student about three years. The student was aghast and asked how long it would take if he spent every possible moment that he could in training. 'That is the easiest question yet!' the Master replied. 'With that attitude, you would never master the art of Tai Chi!'

The point of this story is that so many of the benefits of Tai Chi, and thus the FOF Program, flow from getting the mind and body into a relaxed state. This should be your first objective—the more relaxed your approach to the FOF Program, the better it will work. But, remember a relaxed state means 'dynamic relaxation'—you still have to do things, just make sure that you do them in a relaxed manner!

### WHAT IS THE BEST TIME OF THE DAY TO DO THE EXERCISE MODULE?

The FOF Exercise module can be done just as effectively in the morning, afternoon or evening. Try not to do the Exercise module just after you have eaten. Wait about 30 minutes or more depending on the size of the meal. Also, do not force yourself to exercise when you are feeling hungry, tired or stressed.

The most important thing you can do to ensure the success of your FOF Program is to schedule a fixed time slot for the Exercise module. Experience has shown that if you do the module 'when you have time' you will find that time never materialises and the FOF Program fails before it ever really gets going.

If you can, get a group together to practice the Exercise module. This is very beneficial as it helps to ensure that you will make the time because you do not want to disappoint other members of the group. Somehow that is always more important than disappointing ourselves!

### WHERE IS THE BEST PLACE TO DO THE EXERCISES?

You can perform the Exercise module indoors or out. The best place is anywhere you can exercise undisturbed and the air is fresh. The more pleasant the location, the better you will feel while exercising and the more benefit you will get. Here are some tips to guide you.

- You don't need much space for the FOF Exercise module—only about two square metres of clear space for each person. If you are indoors, for example, you can do the exercises in your lounge room. Alternatively, you could easily find the space outdoors on a veranda or in a garden.
- Make sure that the place you choose for exercising is free from draughts or exposure to damp and extreme heat, cold or wind.
- Take the phone off the hook or turn off the mobile phone. Make it clear to family and friends that they are welcome to join in, but this is your time for your health.

### SHOULD YOU USE MUSIC?

You may find it advantageous to play some relaxing music while you do the FOF exercises. (Avoid anything with a regular beat as such music actually stimulates.) If you like to perform your exercises to the sound of the sea or the sound of water in a fountain or stream, or the breeze in the trees, this would be beneficial, too. Remember that these days you do not need a beach or forest on your doorstep because there are lots of recordings of relaxing natural sound available.

One advantage of playing relaxing music as you exercise is that the subconscious quickly grows to associate the pleasant feelings of relaxation experienced during the exercise session with the music. So, when you play the music at other times, your body will tend to relax even if you are not performing the exercise session. But, equally, don't be surprised when you hear the music if you get the urge to exercise!

In fact, you can use this connection between exercise and music to your own advantage on those days when, for no real reason, you just don't feel like going through the module (yes, it does happen to us all!). Just turn on the music a few minutes before the normal time of your Exercise module and you may suddenly find yourself 'in the mood'.

### WHAT CLOTHING SHOULD YOU WEAR?

As long as your clothing is loose and comfortable, it will suffice. Shoes should be flat-soled.

### WHAT OTHER THINGS CAN IMPROVE THE MODULE?

Access to a mirror may help you check your posture when you do not have an instructor to call your attention to postural defects. A relaxing aroma, such as lavender, can also help you to relax during sessions.

**HOW DO I REMEMBER ALL THE EXERCISES?**

You do not want to be rushing backwards and forwards between the pages of this book during your exercises, so a list of all the exercises is included at the end of this chapter. These pages can be photocopied and put on a wall in front of where you exercise until the sequence becomes familiar to you.

## Set 1 Quiet Standing exercise

Quiet Standing puts you in a relaxed state with proper posture and correct breathing. These are the keys to obtaining the full benefits of Tai Chi or any activity based on Tai Chi such as the FOF Program (see Appendices 1, 2 and 3).

The exercise module starts with Quiet Standing, and we come back to this position after each exercise. We also finish the exercise module with Quiet Standing. Therefore, in the FOF Program, it is used to:

- prepare properly the mind and body for the exercises;e
- provide continuity between each of the sets in the exercise module;
- provide continuity between FOF modules, or prepare for your return in a relaxed state to other activities.

When you perform exercises in this way, you are performing a 'Qigong'—that means that you are working not only with the mind and body but also with the *Chi* or animating energy of the body. In fact, we use this *Chi* energy all the time in everything we do, but, the flow of *Chi* may be blocked or disturbed, for example by incorrect posture or breathing. In traditional Chinese medicine, an excess or deficiency of *Chi* or a disturbance in the flow of this energy is considered to be the source of health problems.

### THE PRACTICE OF QUIET STANDING

To establish the Quiet Standing position, follow these steps in the order that they appear.

- Place your feet shoulder width apart. Your feet should be parallel, with your toes pointing to the front. Try to distribute your weight equally between both feet and centre your balance between your toes and heels. If your weight comes forward on the toes, backward onto the heels or sideways onto one foot or the other, it will cause muscular tension and postural distortion. Check that your toes rest gently on the ground and that they are not clenched or upturned.

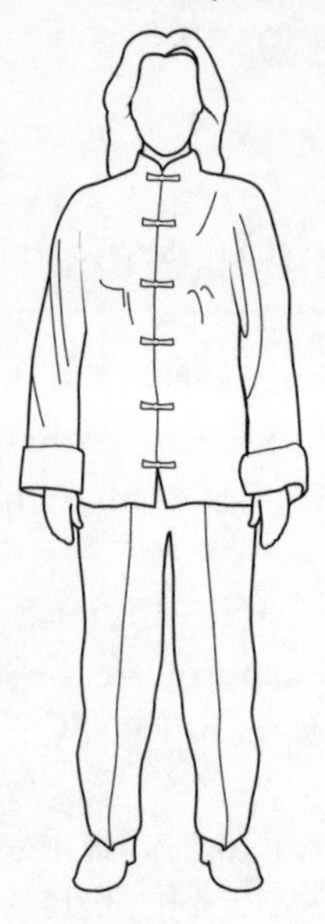

- Imagine that there is a string attached to the crown of your head and your whole body is hanging down from this point with the weight of your body supported by the string. While this step is primarily included to ensure correct physical posture, it is also important from an energetic viewpoint. The point where our 'imaginary' string attaches is the *Bai Hui* acupoint. When we focus our attention on this point, we raise the body's energy and gain a heightened sense of vitality. In Chinese terms, we are 'raising the *shen*'. This effect can be enhanced by feeling that one is 'smiling' through the eyes.

- Now allow yourself to be 'lowered' by the imaginary string until your knees bend naturally into the 'off-lock' position. If this seems difficult, experiment by imagining yourself being alternately raised and lowered by the imaginary string and see how, as you imagine yourself drawn up, your knees seem to straighten without you consciously putting tension into your legs. As you imagine yourself being lowered, your knees will automatically bend and you sink only far enough for your knees to come forward about 2–3 centimetres.

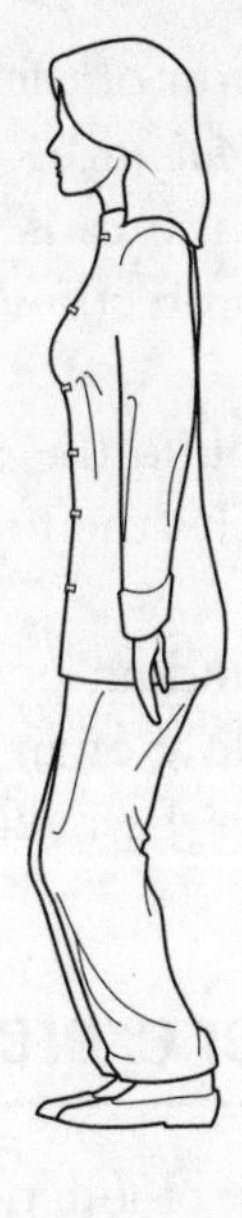

**Sideview; knees in off-lock position**

- Make sure the pelvis is relaxed. Many people tilt the pelvis backwards, causing a pronounced curve in the lumbar area that can lead to many postural distortions and back problems. If you're not sure whether your pelvis is correctly positioned, place your palms over the curve of your pelvic bones, with your thumbs forwards, then tilt your pelvis forward. If you rub the back of one hand down over your lower spine, it should now seem flatter. With the pelvis in the right position, the stomach will tend to feel 'folded'. Despite this sensation, you will find that your pelvis is correctly positioned and relaxed.

- Relax your arms by allowing them to hang loosely at your sides, with your palms facing inward to your body. Then gently lift your shoulders 3–4 centimetres before allowing them to sink down into a comfortable position. As you complete this, stretch your fingertips slowly downwards towards the floor.

- Your mouth should be closed but more through bringing the lips together rather than the teeth. Bringing the teeth together brings tension into the lower jaw. The tip of the tongue can rest against the back of the upper set of teeth or on the hard palate if this is comfortable. Placing the mouth in this position achieves a number of things. Firstly, it ensures that one is breathing through the nose not the mouth. Also, the position of the tongue creates a better connection between the *Du Mai* and *Ren Mai* meridians, the major energy circuits of the body. It also causes increased salivation, which improves both digestion and protection against infection.

- Relax the face, particularly around the eyes (you can do this by slightly tensing the facial muscles then releasing the tension away).

Once you establish the Quiet Standing position, focus on your breath and, with your mind, follow the flow of air into and out of the body at least eight times. Then move on to the next exercise.

## Set 2 Neck and shoulder exercises

The neck is a vital conduit for air, blood, neural messages and *Chi*. It is particularly susceptible to injury and it is important that the muscles in this area remain healthy and free from stress. Unfortunately, the neck musculature is particularly susceptible to stress tensions, particularly those generated from anger and the 'startle reflex' (refer Appendix 1).

People who have had whiplash, 'frozen shoulder' or arthritis in the shoulder or neck area need little persuasion about the importance of this area. However, even they often fail to understand just how much impact this area has on the physical, mental and emotional health of your body.

Try this simple experiment. Raise your shoulders upward and inward towards your ears and hold this position for about one minute or so. Notice the tension building in the back of your neck and the desire to push your head forward?

This tension is an exaggeration of a process that goes on all the time. If your shoulders rise only one-tenth as much as this you carry that tension around all day, you are going to push your head forward. Your head will feel like it weighs as much as a bowling ball, and the result of that weight being thrown forward includes:

- lower back problems as the muscles in this area fight to stop you tipping forward;
- an increased risk of falls as your centre of gravity comes forward;
- curvature of the spine, which compresses the thoracic and abdominal cavities reducing the effective vital capacity of the lungs

(meaning that you breathe faster and shallower, become more anxious, and raise your heart beat and blood pressure);

- postural distortions that, as you walk and move about, cause you to fall forward onto your feet, increasing impact stresses on your ankles, knees, hip joints and the lower vertebra;
- a tendency to spend a lot of time looking at the ground, which has a depressing psychological impact and in turn reduces the efficiency of your immune response;
- an increase in stress levels which impact on the flexibility of the lung diaphragm, aggravating the speed and shortness of breath, reducing blood circulation to the internal organs, and affecting digestion.

And on and on go the cascade of negative effects throughout the body systems—all this from a bit of tension in the shoulders! But, if you look on the bright side, just by getting rid of a little tension in the shoulders, you can make improvements in all these areas!

### WHAT YOU NEED TO KNOW ABOUT THE NECK AND SHOULDER AREA

The joints that we are concerned about in the neck and shoulder area include: the seven cervical vertebrae and the associated musculature for turning and holding those vertebra in place; the ball and socket joints in the shoulders; and the scapulae or shoulder blades. Particularly important are the atlas and axis vertebrae that allow the various movements of the head. These two vertebrae, found at the top of the spine, are the only vertebra that do not have spinal processes. (The spinal processes are anchors for muscle groups, which, in the remainder of the vertebrae, prevent a significant turning movement from side to side.)

The atlas and axis vertebrae are instrumental in generating the significant turning movements that can be achieved by the head. This distinction is important because it means exercises that involve the movement of the head need to be done in a fashion that primarily utilises the atlas and axis vertebrae. If head movements are done in a fashion that over-utilise the five lower neck vertebrae, damage may result.

When considering shoulder movements, we should be careful not to focus simply on the ball and socket joints where the humerus bone connects with the shoulder, but also on the role of the scapulae or shoulder blades. These play a vital part in shoulder movements, being major anchoring points for many of the muscles involved in arm and shoulder movements. Tensions held within the muscles may distort the normal positioning and movement of the shoulder blades.

### RELAXING YOUR JAW

We should not forget the jaw is a joint, too. Many people would say that, with all the eating and talking that goes on, the last thing we need to think about is giving the jaw more exercise! Surprisingly, however, the jaw is an area where considerable tension is stored. This causes problems because the tension:

- reduces the flow of saliva, which is essential for the proper operation of the digestive system;
- impedes the *Chi* energy linkage between the *Du Mai* and *Ren Mai* meridians (the prime *Chi* energy circuits of the body);
- inhibits smiling (and all of its attendant physiological benefits);
- reduces blood supply to gums and teeth, increasing risk of damage and infection;
- can cause grinding of the teeth to the extent of damaging them.

It is therefore important, when breathing in and out through the nose, to bring only the lips together—not the teeth!—and relax your lower jaw.

### DON'T BE DOWNCAST

Shoulder tension has a particularly disturbing effect in that it tends to pull the head forward and downward. Not only does this gradually curve the spine (which compresses the lung cage area, reducing the amount of air that we can breathe and thus affecting our vital energy), but it means that we tend to look downward all the time. This 'downcast' position has particularly adverse affects on our state of mental well-being. Prove it to yourself in this simple little experiment.

Think of a holiday or experience that you really enjoyed. Now, slump your shoulders, bend your neck, and look directly at the floor; describe your holiday or experience. Then, raise your head and look forward, and describe your holiday or experience again. You will notice quite a difference.

### EXERCISING THE NECK SAFELY

The neck is particularly susceptible to injury and damage. Those who have suffered any form of damage to the neck, should secure their doctor's approval before attempting any neck or shoulder exercises. Also:

- do not move your neck in a fast, abrupt movement;
- do not perform neck exercises with your shoulders raised;
- do not continue with any exercise that causes neck pain.

Outside of the FOF Program, if you are performing neck exercises then be alert for the following:

- Avoid any exercise that involves rolling the head in all four directions in sequence. There is too much risk that a moment's loss of focus will result in compaction of neck vertebrae and injury.
- If tilting your head from side to side, do not use hand on your head to increase the stretch. This is unnecessarily dangerous. The same effect will be achieved over time with the weight of the head alone. The danger that you may put excessive strain on the muscles and damage your neck is simply too high to justify.

### THE NECK AND SHOULDER EXERCISES

The exercises for the neck and shoulder area are:

- double shoulder roll
- single shoulder roll
- alternate shoulder roll
- single paddling
- alternate paddling
- shoulder stretch
- horizontal head turns
- vertical head turns
- sideways chin tilts

## DOUBLE SHOULDER ROLL

The benefits of this exercise include removal of tension from the neck and shoulder area, and improvement of blood circulation and of *Chi* in the area. It aids in good posture and the freeing-up of the rib cage with attendant improvements in breathing.

From the Quiet Standing position:

- Roll both the shoulders slowly upward, forward, downward and backward, until they come full circle.

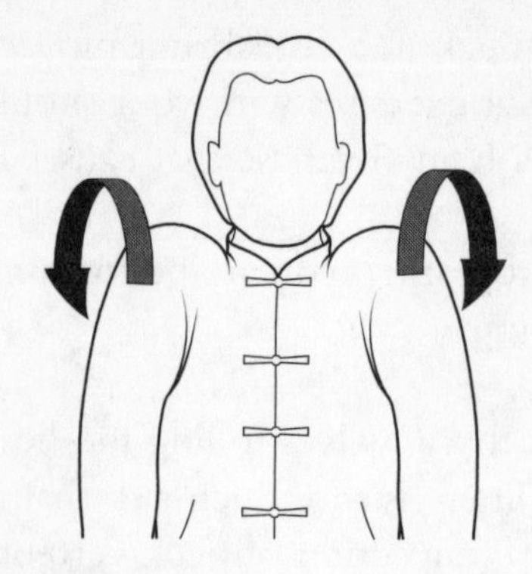

- Repeat to do eight circles. Then reverse the direction of the roll for eight more circles.

***Grandmaster Khor's important points:***

- Do not force the movement or move too fast; look for the smoothness and circularity of the movement. Visualise the area becoming soft and warm.
- Make sure your shoulders do not come inward towards your neck. This is both uncomfortable and tends to increase problems in the area.
- Your arms must remain relaxed. Your shoulders actually lift and lower the arms; you do not use your arms to push up your shoulders. Also, bent elbows are a sign that the arm muscles are being used to force the rotation of the shoulders.
- Your mind should be fully focused on how your shoulder area feels. You should focus on and feel the movement of bone, muscle and sinew. This helps to increase the flow of blood and *Chi*.

**PERFORMING THIS EXERCISE IN QIGONG FORM:**

If you are performing this movement as Qigong, synchronise your breathing as follows:

- Breathe in as you roll your shoulders backward and upward.
- Breathe out as you roll your shoulders forward and downward.

Do not synchronise your breath with the movement unless you are rolling your shoulder slowly—no more than one roll every eight seconds, or you will speed the breathing and inhibit the relaxation response that the Qigong approach is designed to initiate.

## SINGLE SHOULDER ROLL

This movement adds to the benefits of the previous movement because it breaks up muscular tension between the two scapulae or shoulder blades. There is often an incredible amount of tension stored here, with the shoulder blades or scapulae drawn close together. In fact, the shoulder blades of young children are often further apart in relation to those of adults because of this tension!

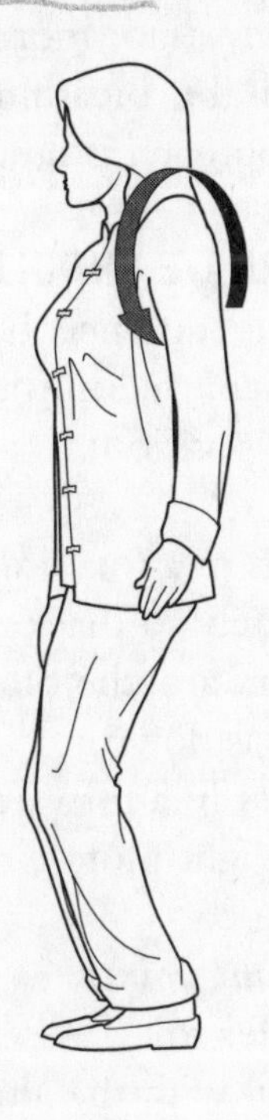

From the Quiet Standing position:

- Roll your right shoulder slowly upward, forward, downward and backward, until it comes full circle.
- Repeat to do four circles. Then reverse the direction of the roll for four more circles.
- Repeat for your left shoulder.

***Grandmaster Khor's important points:***

- As for the double shoulder roll.
- Be aware of the movement between the shoulder blades—one shoulder blade should be rising and falling while the other is still.

**PERFORMING THIS EXERCISE IN QIGONG FORM:**
Synchronise your breathing as follows:

- Breathe in as you roll your shoulder backwards and upwards.
- Breathe out as you roll your shoulder forwards and downwards.

Do not synchronise your breath with the movement unless you are rolling your shoulder slowly—no more than one roll every eight seconds, or you will speed the breathing and inhibit the relaxation response that the Qigong approach is designed to initiate.

## ALTERNATE SHOULDER ROLL

This movement doubles the distance between your shoulder blades compared to that which is achieved in the single shoulder rolls.

From the Quiet Standing position:

- Roll both your shoulders in a forward direction as in the double shoulder roll, but alternately so that one follows the other. That is, when one shoulder is forward, the other is back; when one shoulder is up, the other is down.
- Repeat to do eight circles in a forward direction, then reverse the direction of the roll for eight more circles.

***Grandmaster Khor's important points***

- As for the double shoulder roll.
- Do not be overly forceful with the alternating movement and cause your spine to sway from side to side. Keep your spine upright throughout the movement.

**PERFORMING THIS EXERCISE IN QIGONG FORM**
Synchronise your breathing as follows:

- Breathe in as you roll one shoulder backwards and upwards.
- Breathe out as you roll the same shoulder forwards and downwards.

Do not synchronise your breath with the movement unless you are rolling your shoulders slowly—no more than one roll every eight seconds, or you will speed the breathing and inhibit the relaxation response that the Qigong approach is designed to initiate.

## SINGLE PADDLING

The momentum of the downward movements of the arms pulls the shoulders down, providing a gentle stretch to muscles and ligaments that may be unnaturally shortened due to extended periods of tension.

The movement also helps to remove stress tensions in the shoulders and arms, and improves the circulation of blood and *Chi*.

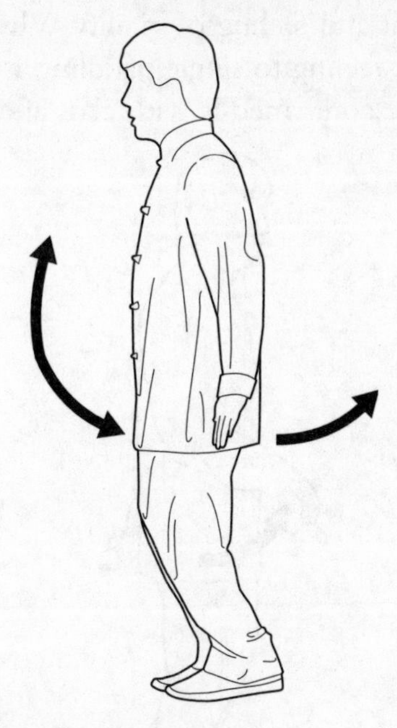

From the Quiet Standing position:

- Swing both your arms gently backwards and forwards, with your palms facing to the back.
- As you bring your hands up to shoulder height, your knees should be in the off-lock position.
- As you bring your hands down, bend your knees and as your hands pass your hips, give your hands a *gentle* flick backwards.
- Continue these movements for about one minute.

***Grandmaster Khor's important points:***

- Ensure you keep your spine upright and your head looking forward throughout the movement. Do not lean forward.

### PERFORMING THIS EXERCISE IN QIGONG FORM

If you are performing this movement as Qigong, do not synchronise it with your breathing or you will breathe too fast and inhibit the relaxation response that the Qigong approach is designed to initiate.

## ALTERNATE PADDLING

This has the same benefits as the previous movement with the additional effect that it is virtually impossible to do this without smiling and getting a real lift to the spirit and feeling of vitality. Why this movement should have such a different feeling to single paddling I have never been able to determine but I have confirmed it with class after class of students.

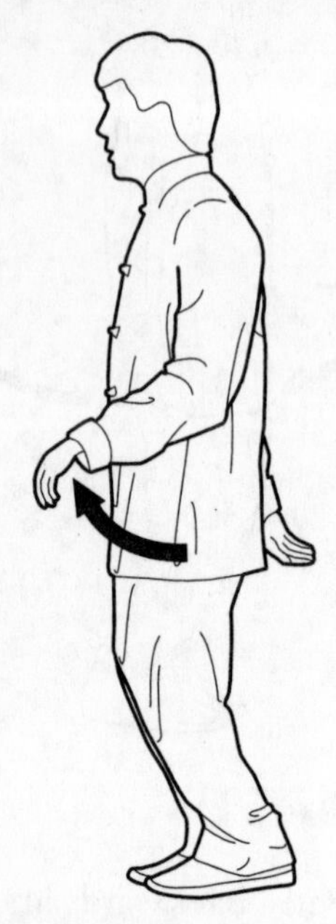

From the Quiet Standing position:

- Repeat the movement for Single Paddling except swing your arms alternately so that one is back while the other is forward.
- As you bring up your right hand to shoulder height, your knees should be in the off-lock position.
- As you bring up your left hand, bend your knees. Continue for about one minute.

***Grandmaster Khor's important points:***
- Make sure that you keep your spine upright and your head looking forward throughout the movement.
- Do not lean forward.

### PERFORMING THIS EXERCISE IN QIGONG FORM

If you are performing this movement as Qigong, do not synchronise it with your breathing or you will breathe too fast and inhibit the relaxation response that the Qigong approach is designed to initiate.

## SHOULDER STRETCH

The movement releases stress tension in the shoulders. Your shoulders will often be noticeably lower after this exercise. It is a useful exercise that can be used to release tension in many situations, even when sitting at a desk.

From the Quiet Standing position:

- Raise your shoulders upward slightly then gently lower them to where they would normally rest.
- Extend your fingertips and push them with a slight pressure downwards (do not force).
- Hold this gentle stretch for the count of four, then slowly release.
- Repeat three times.

***Grandmaster Khor's important points:***
- Move slowly, do not force the movement.
- Your palms should face in to your sides.

### PERFORMING THIS EXERCISE IN QIGONG FORM

If you are performing this movement as Qigong, synchronise your breathing as follows:

- Breathe in as you lift your shoulders to the count of four.
- Breathe out as you lower your shoulders to the count of four
- Breathe in as you stretch downwards to the count of four
- Breathe out as you release the stretch to the count of four.

## HORIZONTAL HEAD TURNS

This movement loosens up and lubricates the axis vertebra and its associated ligaments and muscles. It also strengthens these muscles, thus protecting against injury.

From the Quiet Standing position:

- *Slowly* turn your head from side to side, first looking over your left shoulder and then over your right shoulder.
- Repeat to do the movement four times in each direction.

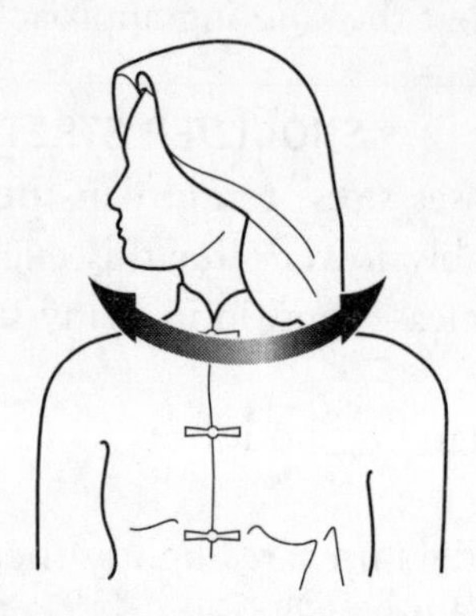

***Grandmaster Khor's important points:***

- Your shoulders should be relaxed and down. If your shoulders start to rise as you turn your head, press your fingers gently downwards.
- Your head should be raised through the *Bai Hui* point. This will help to stretch rather than compact the neck vertebrae (the axis vertebra is the one being exercised).
- The speed of the movement should slow and accelerate naturally at the beginning and end of each turn—there should not be any abrupt change of direction.

**PERFORMING THIS EXERCISE IN QIGONG FORM**

Synchronise your breathing as follows:

- Breathe in as you turn in one direction to the count of four.
- Breathe out as you turn in the other direction to the count of four.

## VERTICAL HEAD RAISES

This movement loosens up and lubricates the atlas vertebra and its associated ligaments and muscles. It also strengthens these muscles, thus protecting against injury.

From the Quiet Standing position:

- *Slowly* tuck in your chin so that you look downwards toward your chest.

- Then slowly lift your chin so that you look upwards toward the sky.
- Repeat to do the movement four times in each direction.

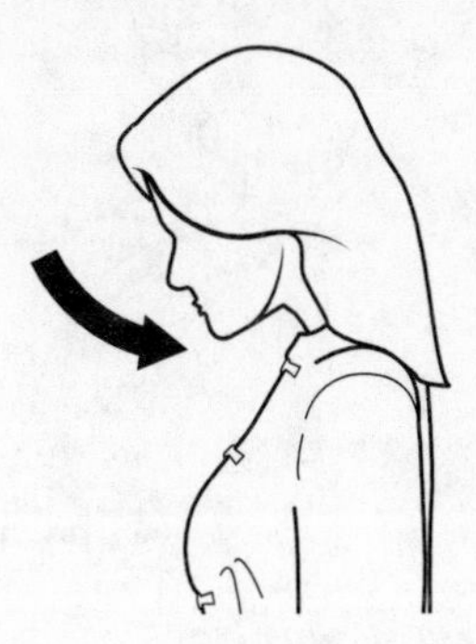

***Grandmaster Khor's important points:***
- Your shoulders should be relaxed and down. If your shoulders start to rise as you turn your head, press your fingers gently downwards.
- Your head should be raised through the *Bai Hui* point. This will help to stretch rather than compact the neck vertebrae (the atlas vertebra is the one being exercised). The movement is like gentle nodding. Do not move the lower five cervical vertebrae either backward or forward.
- The speed of the movement should slow and accelerate naturally at the beginning and end of each move—there should not be any abrupt change of direction.

**PERFORMING THIS EXERCISE IN QIGONG FORM**

If you are performing this movement as Qigong, synchronise your breathing as follows:

- Breathe in as you lift your head upwards to the count of four.
- Breathe out as you lower your head downwards to the count of four.

## SIDEWAYS CHIN TILTS

This movement loosens up and lubricates the atlas vertebra and its associated ligaments and muscles. It also strengthens these muscles, thus protecting against injury.

From the Quiet Standing position:

- Slowly tilt your chin to the left and then to the right.

- Repeat the movement four times in each direction.

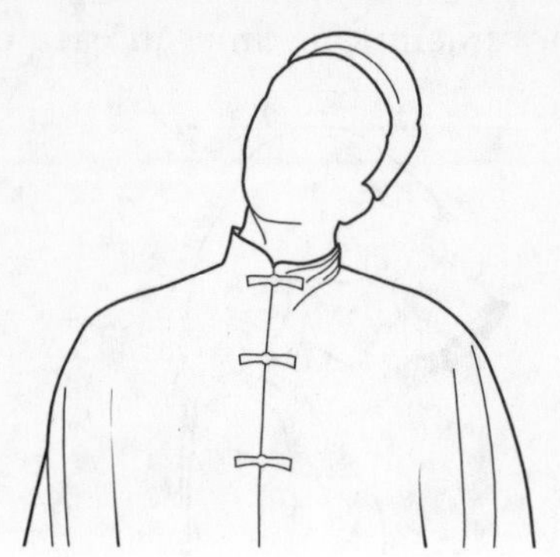

***Grandmaster Khor's important points:***

- Your shoulders should be relaxed and down. If your shoulders start to rise as you tilt your chin, press your fingers gently downwards.
- Your head should be raised through the *Bai Hui* point. This will help to stretch rather than compact the neck vertebrae (the atlas vertebra is the one being exercised). The movement is like gentle nodding. Do not move the lower five cervical vertebrae.
- The speed of the movement should slow and accelerate naturally at the beginning and end of each move—there should not be any abrupt change of direction.

**PERFORMING THIS EXERCISE IN QIGONG FORM**

Synchronise your breathing as follows:

- Breathe in as you tilt your chin in one direction to the count of four.
- Breathe out as you tilt your chin in the other direction to the count of four.

## Set 3 Abdominal exercises

The abdominal cavity houses almost all of the major internal organs including the liver, stomach, pancreas, spleen and kidneys. The abdominal cavity also contains the bulk of the digestive and eliminatory systems so the importance of this area is obvious. What is less obvious is the appropriate types of exercise for this area.

Unfortunately, we tend to store emotional types of stress within the musculature that surrounds the abdominal cavity so relaxation of these muscles is very important. Exercise in this area is not about muscle building, though toning of the abdominal muscles is important. It is about ensuring the removal of tension and the promotion of blood circulation and energy within the abdominal cavity.

### THE ABDOMINAL AREA

The abdominal cavity is separated from the thoracic or chest cavity by a sheet of muscle called the lung diaphragm. It is the downward movement of this muscular sheet that creates the vacuum within the lungs which then draws air into the body. The upward movement of this muscle expels the air. So, if the abdominal area is rigid with tension, this muscular sheet cannot move down and our breathing becomes the short, shallow, stress-response breathing that causes so many problems.

Removing the stress from the abdominal area is not only important for breathing. The upward and downward movement of the lung diaphragm massages the internal organs within the abdominal cavity, squeezing out venous blood on the downward passage and creating negative pressure on the upward movement, encouraging the flow of arterial blood into the internal organs. The massaging effect of the lung diaphragm is also useful for stimulating the intestines and assisting with the passage of food.

There are also sheets of connective tissue that allow the abdominal internal organs to move past each other without injury. If there is little movement in the abdominal area, adhesions begin to develop between these connective tissues and the internal organs and sudden movements may cause these connective tissues to tear. Movement is important to prevent this problem, but do not suddenly perform lots of demanding abdominal exercise. Listen to your body, do not force it.

### THE ABDOMINAL AREA EXERCISES

- Quiet Standing*
- Swinging arms
- Circling the abdomen**
- Kneading the dough
- Drawing in the buttocks

Notes:

* The deep relaxed breathing of Quiet Standing helps to massage the abdominal cavity. If you have already done Quiet Standing as Set 1

of the Exercise module, you do not need to redo this exercise in this part of the program.

★★ Circling the abdomen is a massage technique that, while not strictly an exercise, can be effectively included in the Exercise module instead of the Acumassage module if that is more convenient. (For details of Circling the abdomen, see the Acumassage module.)

## SWINGING ARMS

This movement loosens tensions held in the abdominal muscles, while creating a massaging effect on the internal contents of the abdomen.

From the Quiet Standing position:

- Keeping your back straight, sink your body downwards, feeling as though you are being lowered by a string attached to the crown of your head. Your knees will bend naturally. While you should sink as far as comfortable, do not sink so far that the knees extend in front of the toes. (If you have been too ambitious and the position becomes uncomfortable, slowly rise up and then sink down to a comfortable height.)
- With your arms loose and relaxed at your side, bring your focus to your waist. Using your waist, turn slowly to the left as far as you comfortably can. Do not strain. Keep your body upright.
- Slowly reverse the motion and turn to the right as far as you comfortably can.
- Repeat turning to the left and right, slowly turning faster. With your arms loose and relaxed, you will find that, as you increase speed, your arms will naturally come outwards from your waist and wrap around your body. Just let this happen naturally. There is no pause between the end of one turn and the beginning of another.
- After performing the movement for about two minutes, gradually slow the movement, turning less and less to each side until you come to a gentle stop.

***Grandmaster Khor's important points:***

- To avoid the very common mistake of twisting through the knees, one solution is to use the 'horse-riding stance'. However, one mistake should not be replaced by another, so it is important that your spine remains upright and extended throughout the move.

To ensure that you sink down without spoiling your posture, revert to the image of being supported by a string through the crown of your head and feeling yourself lowered from above. As you sink down into the 'horse-riding stance', visualise that you are pressing your thighs against the horse—the position of your legs will then be more of a U-shape rather than a V-shape.

- Make sure that your body turns through your waist rather than through your knees. Turning your body by twisting your knees has no benefit and may damage your knees. One of the advantages of the 'horse-riding stance' is that it helps to reduce movement in the knees.
- Ensure that your spine remains upright and rotates on its axis rather than twisting from side to side. You can tell whether this is happening or not by visualising that your eyes are painting an imaginary line around the room. The line should be the same height from the floor throughout the whole move. Another indication of a twisting rather than rotating spine is seeing a lot of floor, especially at the end of the turns.
- Keep all tension out of your arms and shoulders.
- Do not stop suddenly at the end of the movement or you will tense the abdominal area.

#### PERFORMING THIS EXERCISE IN QIGONG FORM

If you are performing this movement as Qigong, focus on your posture, keeping your back upright and your shoulders relaxed. Because the movement is relatively fast, do not synchronise your breathing with the movement—just breathe naturally.

### KNEADING THE DOUGH

This movement tones the abdominal muscles and creates a powerful massaging effect on the internal contents of the abdomen. It greatly assists the peristaltic process.

- Stand with your feet shoulder width apart. Keep your back straight and your knees in the off-lock position. Form both hands into fists. Your fists should be held at navel height in front of the body, with the thumb side of the fist upwards and your knuckles at a 45-degree angle to the ground.

- Draw one fist upwards and the other downwards so that they circle each other. Do not create the movement by bending your elbows but rather by using your abdominal muscles.
- Slowly circle the fists 16 times in one direction then 16 times in the other direction.

***Grandmaster Khor's important points:***

- Keep your back straight.
- Do not look down at your fists.
- If you are doing this movement correctly, you will feel a very powerful side-to-side movement in the abdomen. The movement can be surprisingly demanding on the abdominal muscles so don't overdo it the first few times that you practice it.

**PERFORMING THIS EXERCISE IN QIGONG FORM**

If you are performing this movement as Qigong, synchronise your breathing with the drawing up and pushing down of your hands.

## DRAWING IN THE BUTTOCKS

The movement is most beneficial in the lower abdominal area, helping to prevent incontinence. For men, the exercise helps to prevent prostate dysfunction and may be of assistance in some areas of sexual dysfunction.

- Stand with your feet shoulder width apart. Keep your back straight and your knees off-lock.
- Slowly contract the muscles in your buttock area as though you were drawing the anus inwards and upwards.
- Then slowly release the muscular tension.
- Repeat the movement 16 times

***Grandmaster Khor's important points:***

- The movement works on muscles in the buttocks and perineal area that may have become weak so ensure that you do not overdo this movement the first few times that you practice it.
- Practice the movement slowly.

**PERFORMING THIS EXERCISE IN QIGONG FORM**

If you are performing this movement as Qigong, synchronise your inward breath with the tensing of the muscles and your outward breath with the relaxation of the muscles.

## Set 4 Fingers, wrist and elbow exercises

*'Yi dao, Yen dao, So dao'* goes the famous Tai Chi expression. Literally this means 'The way of the mind, the way of the eyes, the way of the hands'. The hands are identified as one of the key Tai Chi elements, yet it is so easy to neglect exercising the joints in this area. The flexibility of our fingers and wrists impacts on the simplest as well as the most complex of our activities.

### WHAT YOU NEED TO KNOW ABOUT THE FINGERS, WRISTS AND ELBOWS AREA

While today's world may have made us more sedentary as a whole, the same cannot be said about our fingers. Many whole body movements have now been replaced by button-pushing actions for our fingers.

Today's activities, such as the use of computer keyboards, have particular impacts on the health of the joints in the fingers and wrists. For instance, I have probably used more than a million key strokes on the computer during the writing of this book alone. Each of those movements was an impact movement for a finger!

We should also be aware that there are 27 bones in each hand and wrist. And that both hands contain more than a quarter of all the bones in our entire body! The area is heavily supplied with nerves because of the fine levels of motor control required in these areas, however, the same concentration of nerves can mean that the fingers and hands can be areas of intense pain when there is localised damage or swelling.

A number of organ meridians extend through the hands and they are part of the major energy circulation of the body so problems in this area can have ramifications across the body. There are, in fact, whole systems of hand reflexology (essentially the stimulation of acupressure points) for treatment of the whole body.

It is very easy to put excess tension into the wrist and fingers (the wrist joint becomes locked and the fingers stiff), or to forget the area entirely (then the wrists become limp and the fingers curled)—I've observed this often in students learning Tai Chi. It is most important that the flow of *Chi* be extended out to the fingertips, but remember that *Chi* will not flow if the area is rigid or tense. People have naturally adopted many techniques for decreasing stress through the stimulation of the hands: worry beads, Baojing balls, pressure balls etc. The hands are often a window to inner turmoil—they fidget and flex, and they are wrung together in situations of high stress.

Note that where there are particular problems with fingers and wrist joints, the hand massage technique from the Acumassage module can be performed just prior to these hand exercises. This improves the circulation and flexibility of the hands and relaxes and removes stress generally.

Baojing ball exercises (see Acumassage module) can also be particularly beneficial for the joints, both directly through exercise of the joints and indirectly through the reduction of stress and the increased flow of blood and *Chi* to the hands. Students with arthritic conditions in the hands who have tried Baojing balls have returned with favourable comments about the improvement of their condition.

**THE FINGERS, WRIST AND ELBOW EXERCISES**

- The golden glove
- Wrist rotations
- Finger flicking
- Turtle swims the ocean
- Presenting the peach

## THE GOLDEN GLOVE

This movement greatly benefits the joints of the hand. The fingers have hinge joints and the flexing of the fingers from the fist to the extended position moves them through these positions. The movement also exercises the bones in the hands between the fingers and wrists.

The visualisation encourages the flow of *Chi* into the hands and the movement will help to remove muscular stress in the hand area.

From the Quiet Standing position:

- Raise your hands in front of your body at about chest height, with your shoulders and elbows relaxed. The palms of your hands face downwards. The fingertips point forward. The thumb is relaxed with the 'tiger's mouth' open but not extended.

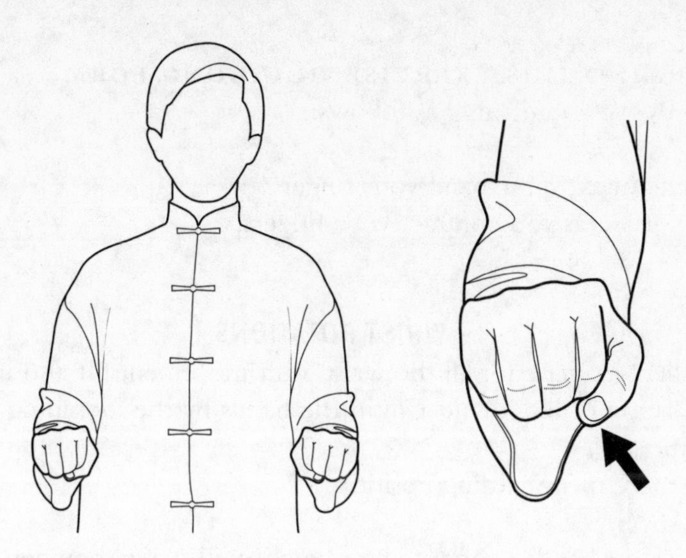

- Slowly form a soft fist with each hand. This is the starting position for the movement.
- Slowly release the fist so that your fingers are again extended with your fingertips pointing directly forward.
- Repeat the movement eight times.

***Grandmaster Khor's important points:***

- Visualisation—imagine your hand is an empty rubber glove attached to a pipe (your arm) that can carry water into and out of the glove. As the glove fills with water, it extends and straightens. As the glove empties, it collapses slowly back into the fist.
- Focus on the 'filling' of your hand rather than stretching. Feel the fullness of the hand. Firstly, it should feel as though the area between the palm and the back of your hand were distending, then the first, second and third segments of the fingers move outwards from the palm.
- To form 'soft fists', your fingers are curled first then the pad of your thumb comes to rest across the second segment of the third finger. The palm is hollow, as though holding a small bird's egg. The strength or tension of the fist is in the third segments of each finger. The 'tiger's mouth' is open.
- As you form the fist, ensure that there is no clenching, just a gentle folding.

**PERFORMING THIS EXERCISE IN QIGONG FORM**

Synchronise your breathing as follows:

- Breathe in as you expand your fingers.
- Breathe out as you contract your fingers.

## WRIST ROTATIONS

An excellent exercise for all the wrist joint movements. It also improves the circulation of blood and *Chi* in the hands by the loosening muscles and ligaments.

From the Quiet Standing position:

- Raise your hands to about chest height with your shoulders and elbows relaxed. The palms of your hands face the ground, fingertips pointing forward. The thumb is relaxed with the 'tiger's mouth' open but not extended. This is the starting position for this movement.
- Rotate your wrists so that your fingertips move in circles in an anticlockwise direction. Complete eight circles.
- Rotate your wrists so that your hands move in a clockwise direction. Complete eight circles.
- Bring your hands back down to your side.

***Grandmaster Khor's important points:***

- Keep all tension out of your hands.
- Avoid causing any pain but do not worry about lots of cracking and clicking that might occur.
- Make sure that the elbows remain still. This can be checked by grasping the wrist of that hand with the other while circling one hand. It is also a good time to feel the amount of movement that occurs in tendons and muscles when this exercise is performed.

## FINGER FLICKING

This movement gets the blood and *Chi* out to your fingertips. It also loosens muscular tensions in your hands. It is a good exercise for the hand joints, particularly the fingers.

From the Quiet Standing position:

- Form soft fists at about heart height and hold your firsts about shoulder width apart.
- Flick your fingers and thumbs apart, as though you are flicking water off your fingers. Your elbows should remain still with all the movement coming from you wrist and fingers.
- Repeat the movement 16 times.

***Grandmaster Khor's important points:***

- Keep the 'flicking' continuous.
- Do not synchronise with your breathing.

**PERFORMING THIS EXERCISE IN QIGONG FORM**

If you are performing this movement as Qigong, maintain posture with relaxed shoulders and elbows. Do not synchronise your breathing with the movement as you will raise your breathing rate too high.

## TURTLE SWIMS THE OCEAN

This movement provides good exercise for the elbows while also working on the wrists and shoulder joints.

From the Quiet Standing position:

- Raise your arms to shoulder height, with your hands shoulder width apart. Your fingertips should point forward, your palms face outwards. Your shoulders, elbows and wrists should be relaxed.

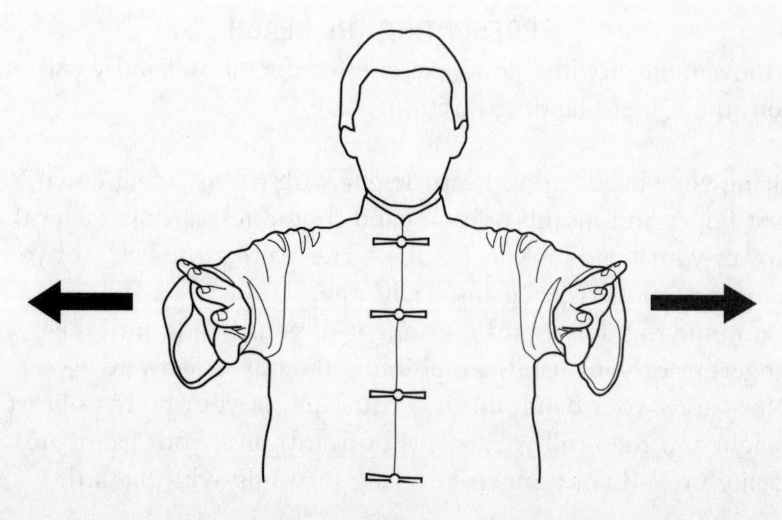

- Sweep your hands outwards, backwards and downwards to about hip height. Continue the movement of your hands so that they come inwards towards the body, with your fingertips pointing forwards and your palms facing up, at hip height on each side.
- Thrust your hands forward until they are again at shoulder height then turn your palms outward and repeat four times.
- Now reverse the direction of the movement, drawing your palms inwards and downwards to hip height on either side of the body. Turn your wrist so that your fingertips point to the back, keep your palms facing up.
- Push your arms backwards and outwards until they return to shoulder height in front of the body and repeat four times.

***Grandmaster Khor's important points:***
- Keep your shoulders relaxed throughout.

### PERFORMING THIS EXERCISE IN QIGONG FORM

If you are performing this movement as Qigong, maintain posture with relaxed shoulders and elbows. Synchronise your breathing as follows:

- Breathe out as you thrust your hands forward.
- Breathe in as you sweep your hands from front to back.
- Breathe in as you draw your hands inwards in reverse motion.
- Breathe out as you sweep your hands from back to front.

## PRESENTING THE PEACH

This movement provides good exercise for the elbows and wrist joints.
From the Quiet Standing position:

- Bring your hands up to heart height with palms facing down. Your first finger and thumb of each hand should rest against each other. Lower your hands as you roll the wrists so that the backs of your hands and fingers lie against each other.
- Continue the downward movement of your hands until the fingertips of your hands are pointing directly downward.
- Now, draw your hands up the centre line of your body to heart height and then roll your wrists outwards until your palms are facing up and your fingertips facing forwards, with the little

fingers of each hand lying against each other.

- Roll your hands inwards until the palms face down, with the sides of the thumbs and first fingers touching each other again.
- Do the movement eight times for forward and reverse directions.

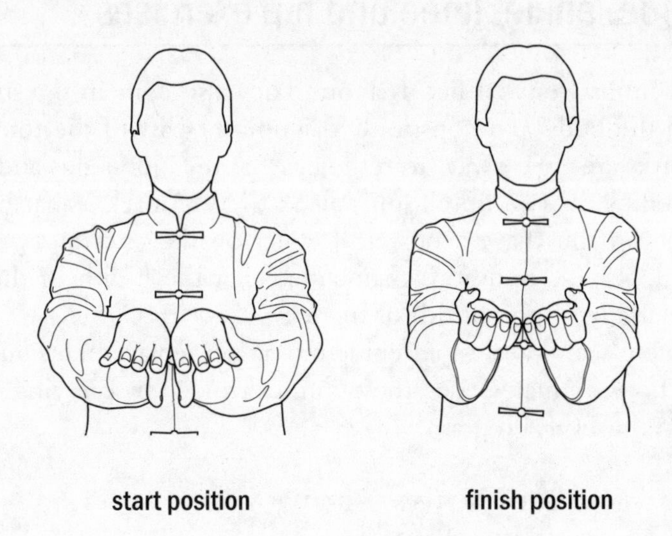

start position          finish position

***Grandmaster Khor's important points:***

- Keep your shoulders relaxed.
- Move slowly.

**PERFORMING THIS EXERCISE IN QIGONG FORM**

Maintain your posture with relaxed shoulders and elbows. Synchronise your breathing with the movement as follows:

- Breathe in as you bring your hands downward and inward.
- Breathe out as you bring your hands upward and outward.
- Breathe in as you bring your hands inward and downward in reverse motion.
- Breathe out as you bring your hands upward and outward.

If you visualise yourself drawing energy into the *Tan Tien* as you bring your hands downward and inward and then taking the energy up the centre line of the body and out from the heart, the exercise can be particularly useful in releasing heart energy that has accumulated as emotional tension around the heart area. The reverse motion will also wash energy through this area but it should be done only after the release motion.

## Set 5 Toe, ankle, knee and hip exercises

The lower limbs are what get us about. They also contain the strongest muscles in the body and constitute a significant part of the total body mass. The feet are as far away from the heart as the blood gets and, when we are standing, it is an uphill journey all the way back. What happens in the legs can thus have a powerful effect on the circulatory system. Indeed the Chinese traditions maintained that the health of the body depended largely on the health of the legs.

Today there seems almost an epidemic of hip replacements and knee reconstructions. In many cases, these can be avoided by carrying out the activities in the FOF Program.

### WHAT YOU NEED TO KNOW ABOUT YOUR TOES, ANKLES, KNEES AND HIPS

There a number of things that you need to know about how your feet and legs function if you are going to maintain their health and function.

The hip joint is a ball and socket joint, with considerable range of movement. Unfortunately, as we get older and more sedentary, we tend to use only a limited degree of movement in the hip joint. Degeneration of the joint sets in and before we know it we are marking the date of that hip replacement in our calendar. The hip joint needs to be regularly and fully rotated through its full range of movements.

The knee joint has the reverse problem. We use it for things that we shouldn't. Our muscles get lazy as we stand so we lock our knees back, taking the weight of the body on the joint and reducing blood circulation in the area. The heavier we are, the worse the problem. The less we exercise the leg muscles, the worse the problem. Treat the knee like this too often and you can pencil in a knee reconstruction next to the hip replacement.

Leonardo da Vinci was overawed by the architectural brilliance of the design of the foot. We treat them like blocks of wood on the end of our legs when the feet are indeed a marvellous design. As you step forward with a foot, the bones lock into place to provide a firm anchor for the muscles to propel the body forward. As the same foot is lifted, the interlocking bone structure relaxes, the blood and body fluids flow into the foot to nourish it. When the foot reaches the ground, it is full of fluid and the bone structure is relaxed so the foot can easily absorb the shock of impact. If you carry tension in the foot and lower leg, all this changes. The bone structure remains locked, the foot does not get the proper supply of fluid to provide nutrients for its health and to absorb the shock of impact. This impact can damage the foot or travel upwards through the body to damage the knee, hip or lower vertebra. This is one reason why jogging can be so dangerous if performed with poor posture or on a hard surface.

Finally, we must realise is that the knee is basically a hinge joint. It has a limited range of movements in other directions, but these are best used when that particular leg is not holding up the body's weight. When the leg is under load and the knee moves in a different direction to the ankle, there is a shearing stress on the knee that, if repeated often enough, will damage the knee. Unfortunately, one of the effects of muscular stress in the hip area is too turn the leg outwards, causing the toes to also face slightly outwards as we walk, and creating that very shearing stress on the knee that we are so concerned with.

The objectives of the FOF Program are therefore to:

- remove stress from the muscles in the legs;
- keep the leg musculature well toned;
- use proper body mechanics when moving.

### TOES, ANKLES, KNEES AND HIPS EXERCISES

- Walking on the spot
- Knee and ankle rotations
- Circling the knee
- Circling the ankle
- Hip rotation
- Cross-legged sit
- Tai Chi walking

## WALKING ON THE SPOT

This movement benefits the joints by exercising the hinge joints in the ankles and toes. The turning of the knee inwards and outwards exercises the ball and socket joint in the hip. It is also quite a good cardiovascular exercise that helps to develop muscle tone.

From the Quiet Standing position:

- Shift your weight onto your right foot and lift your left knee as high as possible while leaving the left toes in contact with the ground.
- Lower your left knee so all of your left foot is in contact with the ground and then shift all of your body weight onto your left foot.
- Lift your right knee as high as possible while leaving your right toes in contact with the ground.
- Lower your right knee so all of your right foot is on the ground.
- Repeat the movement sequence for about one minute.
- Now, do the movement but each time you lift a knee, turn it outwards as far as comfortable. Then turn it back to face forward and lower the knee as before. Repeat this four times on each side.
- Finally, do the movement but each time you lift a knee, turn it inwards as far as comfortable. Then turn it back to face forward and lower the knee as before. Repeat this four times on each side.

***Grandmaster Khor's important points:***

- The base of the toes must remain on the ground. This allows your foot to flex.
- Your upper body should be relaxed, with your arms hanging freely at the sides.
- Keep your posture upright, looking straight ahead rather than down at your feet.
- When your knee is lifted, your foot should rest on the ground free of tension but keep your weight off this foot.
- The knee of the supporting leg should be in the off-lock position.

## KNEE AND ANKLE ROTATIONS

This movement benefits the joints by loosening up the knee, ankle and hip. It also strengthens muscle tone in the legs, improves balance, and reduces stress tensions in the lower part of the body.

From the Quiet Standing position:

- Open your left foot so that your left knee and toes point outward from the body at about 45 degrees.

- Shift the weight of your body to your left leg, bending your left knee slightly.
- Lift your right leg and place the large toe of your right foot on the ground, with your heel lifted.
- Move your right knee in a vertical circle in a clockwise direction eight times.
- Move your right knee in a vertical circle in an anticlockwise direction eight times.
- Bring the position back into the Quiet Standing posture.
- Then repeat the above steps, shifting the weight of your body to your right leg and circling your left knee.

***Grandmaster Khor's important points:***

- Make sure the knee on the supporting leg is kept bent in the off-lock positions so that your body weight is held by the muscles and not by a locked knee joint.
- Keep your posture upright, looking straight ahead not down at the circling knee.

#### PERFORMING THIS EXERCISE IN QIGONG FORM

If you are performing this movement as Qigong, breathe naturally but ensure that a balanced, upright posture is maintained.

### CIRCLING THE KNEE

This exercise frees up the movement of the knee joint. The weight of the lower leg hanging from the knee provides a gentle stretch to the knee ligaments. It also relaxes the foot and lower leg muscles and tendons, builds up muscle tone in the legs, and improves balance and coordination.

From the Quiet Standing position:

- Open your left foot so that your left knee and toe point outward from your body at about 45 degrees.
- Shift the weight of your body to your left leg, bending your left knee slightly.
- Lift your right leg so that the upper leg is parallel to the ground, with the lower leg hanging without any part of the foot touching the ground. (Those who have difficulty with this should lean against a wall or chair.)

- Move your right foot in horizontal circles in a clockwise direction four times. Move in an anticlockwise direction four times.
- Return to the Quiet Standing position.
- Then repeat the above steps with your weight on your right leg and with your left foot circling.

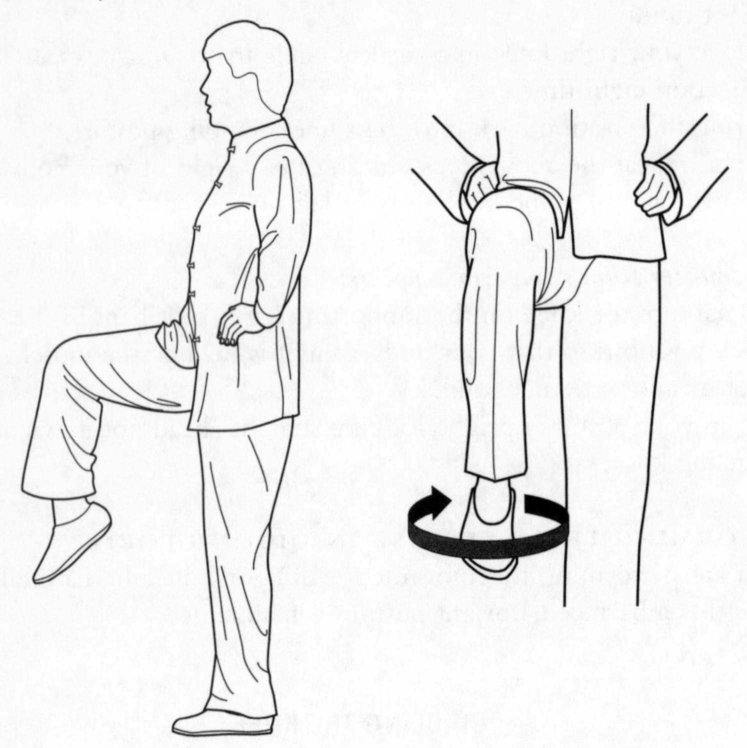

***Grandmaster Khor's important points:***

- Make sure that the knee on the supporting leg is kept slightly bent so that your body weight is held by the muscles and not by a locked knee joint.
- Keep your posture upright, looking straight ahead and not down at the circling knee.
- Allow the circling foot to hang loosely. Circle with the sole of your foot rather than the toes, otherwise there will be tension in your foot. If it helps, you can imagine there is a pencil projecting from the centre of the sole of your foot. If this were in contact with a sheet of paper on the ground, it would trace a circle on that paper.
- Make the movements smooth slow and even. There is often a

tendency to rush this movement because of balance problems. It is better to support yourself on a wall or chair than to be constantly whipping back and forth in order to balance.

#### PERFORMING THIS EXERCISE IN QIGONG FORM

If you are performing this movement as Qigong, breathe naturally but ensure that a balanced upright posture is maintained.

### CIRCLING THE ANKLE

This exercise frees up the movement of the ankle and toe joints. The weight of the lower leg hanging from the knee provides a gentle stretch to the knee ligaments. It also relaxes the foot and lower leg muscles and tendons, builds up muscle tone in the legs, and improves balance and coordination.

From the Quiet Standing position:

- Open your left foot so that your left knee and toe point outwards from the body at about 45 degrees.
- Shift the weight of your body to your left leg, bending your left knee slightly.
- Lift your right leg so that the upper leg is parallel to the ground, with the lower leg hanging without any part of the foot touching the ground. (Those who have difficulty with this should lean against a wall or chair.)
- Move the toes of your right foot in vertical circles in a clockwise direction four times.

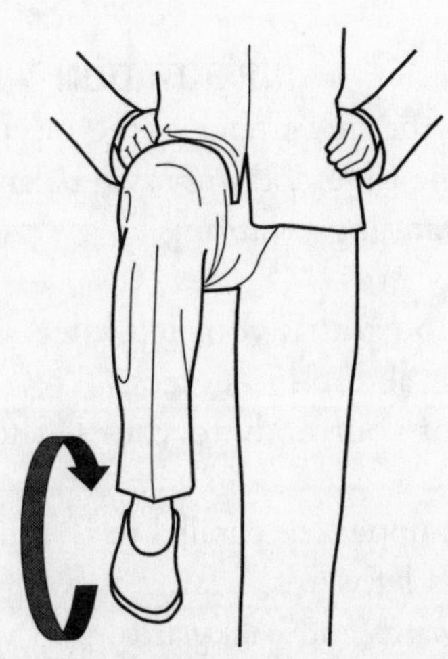

- Move the toes of your right foot in vertical circles in an anticlockwise direction four times.
- Return to the Quiet Standing posture.
- Repeat the above steps with your weight on your right leg and with your left foot circling.

***Grandmaster Khor's important points:***

- Make sure that the knee on the supporting leg is kept bent so that your body weight is held by the muscles and not by a locked knee joint.
- Keep your posture upright, looking straight ahead and not down at the circling foot.
- Allow the circling foot to hang loosely. Circle with the sole of your foot rather than the toes, otherwise there will be tension in your foot. If it helps, imagine there is a pencil projecting from the centre of the sole of your foot. If this were in contact with a sheet of paper on the ground, it would trace a circle on that paper.
- Make the movements smooth, slow and even. There is often a tendency to rush this movement because of balance problems. It is better to support yourself on a wall or chair than to be constantly whipping back and forth in order to balance.

#### PERFORMING THIS EXERCISE IN QIGONG FORM

If you are performing this movement as Qigong, breathe naturally but ensure that a balanced upright posture is maintained.

## HIP ROTATION

This exercise frees up the movement of the hip joints. It also relaxes these joints, builds up muscle tone, and improves balance and coordination.

From the Quiet Standing position:

- Open your left foot so that your left knee and toe point outward from your body at about 45 degrees.
- Shift the weight of your body to your left leg, bending your left knee slightly.
- Keeping the right upper leg parallel to the ground, move your right knee outwards and leftwards as far as is comfortable. Now push your right knee downwards and backwards until your right leg is

extended with the toes of your right foot resting on the ground. Then bring your right knee upwards and forwards until your right upper leg is again parallel to the ground. Repeat four times.

- Now reverse the above steps by pushing the knee downwards and backwards until your right leg is extended behind your body, with your toes touching the ground. Rotate your knee outwards then lift your knee so that the upper leg is parallel with the ground. Arc your knee inwards, keeping the upper leg parallel to the ground, until the hip joint is fully closed. Repeat four times.
- Return to the Quiet Standing position.
- Repeat the entire movement with your weight on your right leg and with the left hip joint rotating.

***Grandmaster Khor's important points:***

- Make sure the knee on the supporting leg is kept bent so your body weight is held by muscles and not by a locked knee joint.
- Keep your posture upright, looking straight ahead and not down at your knee.

#### PERFORMING THIS EXERCISE IN QIGONG FORM

If you are performing this movement as Qigong, breathe naturally but ensure that a balanced upright posture is maintained.

### CROSS-LEGGED SIT

This movement provides a good stretch for the ligaments and tendons around the knee area. It is also a significant strengthening exercise for the leg muscles.

From the Quiet Standing position:

- Open your left foot so that your left toes and knee point outwards from your body at about 45 degrees.
- Shift the weight of your body to your left leg and, with your right leg, step behind and slightly to the left of your left leg.
- Keeping your weight on your left leg and your body upright, lower your body as far as comfortable by bending your knees.
- Raise your body by using your leg muscles to straighten your legs back into the off-lock position.
- Shift the weight of your body to your right leg and, with your left

leg, step behind and slightly to the right of your right leg.

- Repeat the above steps and step back slowly, leaning enough to the left so that your right foot comes slightly off the floor.
- Now, keeping your weight on your right leg and your body upright, lower your body as far as comfortable by bending your knees.
- Raise your body by using your leg muscles to straighten your legs back into the off-lock position.
- Repeat the entire movement four times.
- Then return to the Quiet Standing position.

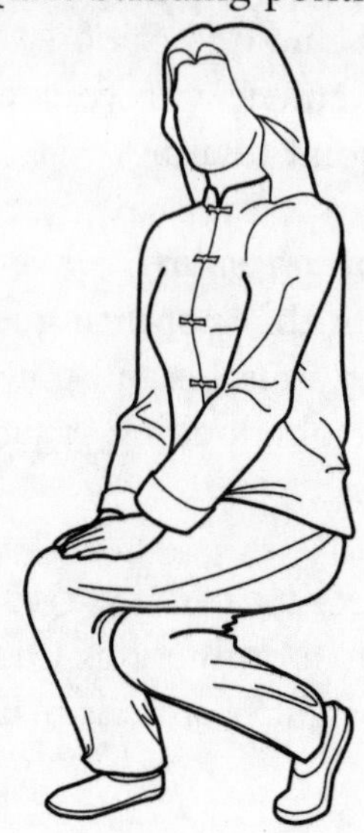

***Grandmaster Khor's important points:***

- Make sure that the knee on the supporting leg is kept off-lock so that your body weight is held by the muscles and not by a locked knee joint.
- Keep posture upright, look straight ahead and not at the legs.
- Sink only as far as comfortable and no further than a level that brings your upper leg parallel with the ground. (It is possible to sink lower but the leverage loading on the knee rises dramatically to be potentially dangerous.) If you wish to improve your strength, it is better to increase the number of times you sink rather than the depth to which you sink.
- If you have difficulty in rising, use your hands to press down on your upper legs.

- Make the movements smooth slow and even. If there is any sharp pain during this exercise, discontinue immediately and seek medical advice before attempting to proceed.

### PERFORMING THIS EXERCISE IN QIGONG FORM

Breathe out as you sink and breathe in as you rise. Ensure that a balanced, upright posture is maintained.

## TAI CHI WALKING

The different elements of this movement have the following benefits:

- Moving with the knees bent tones the muscles and protects the joints, while stimulating the cardiovascular system.
- Facing the toes forward as you step protects the knee joint and helps to remove muscular tensions in the abdominal area.
- Keeping the feet shoulder width apart increases stability and reduces the risk of falls.
- Relaxing the raised foot ensures health of the feet through improved circulation and improves the venous blood return system in the legs. It also allows the bone structure to realign for the re-impact of the foot, protecting the foot, joints and spine.

From the Quiet Standing position:

- Transfer your weight to your left leg and open your right toe at 45 degrees to your body.
- Transfer your weight to your right leg, slowly lifting your left knee until your left foot is clear of the ground.
- Slowly extend your left foot forward and lower your left knee until the heel touches the ground.
- As you transfer your weight to your left foot, bring your left foot into full contact with the ground.
- Transfer your weight to your right leg and open your left foot at 45-degree angle to your body.
- Transfer your weight to your left leg, slowly lifting your right knee until your right foot is clear of the ground.
- Slowly extend your right foot forward and lower your right knee until the heel touches the ground.

- As you transfer your weight to your right foot, bring your right foot into full contact with the ground.
- Repeat the entire movement eight times.

***Grandmaster Khor's important points:***

- Keep your knees bent at all times. Particularly watch the tendency to straighten the supporting leg as you step forward. If anything, you should sink slightly on this leg as you raise the other leg.
- The foot of the raised leg should be kept relaxed and allowed to hang naturally.
- When you step forward, keep that foot about a shoulder width from the supporting foot. The toes should point directly forward, not to the side.
- Do not step too far forward. (As a test, you should be able to lower the whole foot onto the floor without transferring any weight.)
- Separate the placing of the foot from the transfer of weight. (As a test, you should be able to move your foot backwards and forwards without any transfer of weight.)
- Transfer your weight by using your knees together, rather than by 'bouncing' up and down as occurs when you bend your knees independently.
- Keep your back straight and your tailbone tucked under.
- Keep your leg movements slow and smooth.

#### PERFORMING THIS EXERCISE IN QIGONG FORM

If you are performing this movement as Qigong, synchronise your breathing as follows:

- Breathe in as you move your weight back to open the toe.
- Breathe out as you step forward and transfer your weight forward.

# Summary of exercises

**SET 1 QUIET STANDING EXERCISE**

- The practice of quiet standing

**SET 2 NECK AND SHOULDER EXERCISES**

- Double shoulder roll
- Single shoulder roll
- Alternate shoulder roll
- Single paddling
- Alternate paddling
- Shoulder stretch
- Horizontal head turns
- Vertical head raises
- Sideways chin tilts

**SET 3 ABDOMINAL EXERCISES**

- Swinging arms
- Kneading the dough
- Drawing in the buttocks

**SET 4 FINGERS, WRIST AND ELBOW EXERCISES**

- The golden glove
- Wrist rotations
- Finger flicking
- Turtle swims the ocean
- Presenting the peach

**SET 5 TOE, ANKLE, KNEE AND HIP EXERCISES**

- Walking on the spot
- Knee and ankle rotations
- Circling the knee
- Circling the ankle
- Hip rotation
- Cross-legged sit
- Tai Chi walking

Part 3

# The FOF Program Breathing and Meditation Module

# The Breathing and Meditation Module

MEDITATION MEANS NO MORE than to focus or be aware of a particular sound, sight, sensation or activity. In other words, to have the mind and the body's senses focused on the same object. For the meditation process to be beneficial, we need to focus on something that is pleasant and engaging. Few people would achieve positive results when meditating on the sound of chalk squeaking across a blackboard, a vile taste or odour, or the sight of a garbage tip.

Some people presume that to meditate is to think about nothing, but this is actually a contradiction in terms. If you were told to not think about a green horse, the only way you could be sure that you had not thought about a green horse would be to review the contents of your mind for the mental image of a green horse! Replace the words 'green horse' with 'nothing' and the contradiction becomes more apparent.

Thinking of 'nothing' is actually directed meditation; it is not non-thinking. This is not to say that we cannot meditate on the 'sensation' of a calm, quiet mind, letting go of thoughts as they enter our mind. Many people go to sleep when they try to practice 'non-thinking'. They are focusing on turning off the conscious mind and they succeed. This can be overcome by practicing standing meditation. Other people, who remain awake, become frustrated that their conscious mind exhibits its consciousness by retaining a state of awareness, with distracting thoughts continually drifting across their mind. Such meditation is not likely to be perceived as relaxing and, in fact, can be quite stressful.

We know that meditation:

- changes the brainwaves that are produced in the mind to the pleasant and healthy alpha pattern;
- induces the 'relaxation response' that puts the body into its growth and repair mode;
- plays a similar role to sleep in refreshing and reinvigorating the body.

I WILL ALWAYS REMEMBER PICKING UP A PLAQUE WITH THE INJUNCTION THAT ONE SHOULD:

'PERFECT THE ART OF TAKING MINUTE VACATIONS.'

Some interesting studies in the United States have shown that people who meditated regularly tended to have a state of health that was associated with people five to 12 years younger than their chronological age. Meditation can also improve concentration, emotional stability, and the capacity to enjoy life!

The history of meditation probably goes back as long as man's mind has been conscious. The ancient Chinese developed their own unique approach. First, they focused on the fact that the mind had two parts (these days, in the West, we now refer to this as the 'right' and 'left' brain functions). In Chinese terms, this was an aspect of the *Yin–Yang* nature of the universe. The *Yin* part of the mind, the '*shen*', dealt with emotion and feeling and was the source of intuition and creativity. The *Yang* part of the mind, the '*Yi*', dealt with logical, rational thought and involved intellect, memory and willpower. Chinese meditation was about developing and harmonising both these parts through directed activity.

One form of direction that has many benefits is *Chi* meditation. This is a technique for moving the *Chi* around the body using the mind. Since the free flow of *Chi* is the basis of our health and energy, developing skills in this area can be very valuable. Other meditation techniques based on sound and colour are also included as methods most useful for particular healing objectives. We also look at the bone breathing technique, a powerful meditation form particularly useful for developing strong healthy bones. Finally we look at the role of positive thinking.

Meditation shouldn't be a big deal, but a normal natural part of everyday life. The simpler things are often better. You might also make meditation a part of your life by taking a break and stopping to admire a view, pat a dog, relive a beautiful memory, savour a food and so on. There is great wisdom to be found in this approach to life.

### HOW LONG SHOULD EACH TECHNIQUE TAKE?

Unless there are medical reasons to the contrary, you should try to meditate for continuous periods of 20 minutes or more so that the relaxation response is initiated.

### HOW OFTEN AND WHEN SHOULD THIS MODULE BE DONE?

There is no fixed requirement for meditation per week. If you spent 20 minutes each day meditating, this would be more than adequate.

The Breathing and Meditation module can be done just as effectively in the morning, afternoon or evening. Avoid times when you will be disturbed by interruptions and try to meditate on your own.

### WHERE IS THE BEST PLACE TO DO THIS MODULE?

The location should be one where there is good circulation of air and no extreme environmental factors such as heat, cold, strong wind, noise, excessive movement of people or vehicles. The more pleasant the environment in terms of comfort, view, quality of air and quality of sound, the better the meditation results will be.

### SHOULD YOU USE MUSIC IN THIS MODULE?

Music can assist your meditation if it is the focus of the meditation. In such instances, the music should not have a beat nor should it be overly complex. Bamboo flute music, Koto music, or the sound of bells as well as other simple sounds can all be beneficial.

### WHAT CLOTHING SHOULD YOU WEAR FOR THIS MODULE?

As long as clothing is loose and comfortable, it will suffice.

**ARE THERE ANY OTHER THINGS THAT IMPROVE THE BENEFITS OF THE MODULE**

A relaxing aroma, such as lavender, can help you to relax during meditation. Pine and lemon aromas can stimulate and refresh the mind.

## The Techniques for the breathing and meditation module

- Technique 1 *Chi* meditation
- Technique 2 Golden cloud meditation
- Technique 3 Colour meditation
- Technique 4 Sound meditation
- Technique 5 Bone breathing meditation
- Technique 6 Positive thinking
- Technique 7 Smiling

This module also uses the breathing techniques detailed in Appendix 3.

# Technique 1 *Chi* meditation

The meditation systems of some cultures view the body as a distracting nuisance that had to be ignored or dominated, but, the ancient Chinese thought more in terms of a body–mind relationship, rather than a separate mind and body (for instance, the emotional aspects of '*shen*' were based on the energetic condition of various organ systems). Therefore the body is an integral part of the meditative process. And, as a result, *Chi* meditation techniques are actually body–mind meditative techniques that pay attention to all aspects of the body, be they physical, energetic, intellectual or emotional.

*Chi* meditation is based on an understanding of how *Chi* flows within the body, and these can be very complex. However, the meditation techniques themselves can be practiced with only a basic knowledge of the *Chi* flow, storage and transformation process.

For those who have not yet experienced the sensations and effects of *Chi* flow, the fact that the mind has the ability to move the *Chi* around the body should not really be so surprising—even the august publication *Scientific American* has reported experiments where the simple act of focusing the mind on a beaker of water succeeded in creating a measurable rise in the temperature of the water.

### BREATHING AND *CHI* MEDITATION

Breathing is a most important aspect of *Chi* meditation—it helps to focus and direct the *Chi* energy. There are a number of breathing techniques that can be used but the best way to start is with the use of diaphragmatic breathing (see Appendix 3).

### VISUALISATION AND *CHI* MEDITATION

Visualisation is a process that is used to lead the flow of *Chi* energy by focusing on acupoints, meridians and particular mental imagery.

### POSTURE AND *CHI* MEDITATION

There are many *Chi* meditation postures, including Quiet Standing (*see* Exercise module) and Quiet Sitting (*see* below). (Also *see* Appendix 2.) Each posture has its own advantages, but note that no reference has been made to lying down or prone postures. There are many reasons for this.

The major *Chi* circulation system in the body consists of the *Du Mai* and *Ren Mai* meridians. The circulation of *Chi* within this system is maximised when the spine is vertical and extended, as though the head is lifted through the crown of the skull. The coccyx should also be tucked under. This is very difficult to achieve in a lying position. Further, especially when lying flat on the back, the internal organs are incorrectly positioned—the contents of the abdominal cavity press back against the diaphragm and inhibit proper breathing. The *Chi* circulation system is, if anything, hard to properly activate lying down.

Note, too, that kneeling and lotus-type postures, where one sits cross-legged, can also cause problems by cutting off the circulation of *Chi* energy, especially if you are unfamiliar with the position.

## QUIET SITTING POSTURE

- Choose a stool or chair. Make sure it is the correct height—when you sit with the base of your spine close to the front edge of the stool or chair, your feet should rest comfortably on the floor, with your upper leg horizontal and your lower leg vertical. If using a chair, the seat should be firm and should not slope backwards.
- Sit on the front third of the seat. Your spine should be maintained in an upright position.
- Your feet should be placed flat on the ground, about shoulder width apart, with the feet parallel and toes pointing to the front.

Your upper legs should be horizontal and the lower legs perpendicular, so that the small amount of weight resting on the legs is equally placed on both feet and equally distributed over the heel and base of the toes.

- Your head should feel as though lifted by a string from the centre of the top of the head (the *Bai Hui* acupoint). Your jaw should be relaxed and tucked slightly inwards and downwards.
- Your shoulders and elbows should be relaxed, with your palms resting on the upper thighs. Your fingertips are gently extended and the tiger's mouth (the area between the thumb and first finger) is open. Make sure that your shoulders are at equal height and face forward, preventing bowing or twisting of the spine.
- Your chest and abdomen should be relaxed and spine straight.
- Your eyes are relaxed and looking straight ahead. Rather than looking at something, let whatever is in front of you come to you. This will prevent you focusing too strongly.
- Keep your lips gently together but the teeth separated, with the tip of your tongue resting on the upper palate.
- Now move on to the mental posture.
- Relax and focus your mind on the *Chi Hai* point. Imagine yourself breathing down to this point and out to the tip of the nose. Make sure your abdomen feels relaxed and feel it moving outwards with each in-breath and inwards with each out-breath.
- After you have established your breathing pattern, focus your mind on your body and observe what happens each time you breathe to your shoulders, chest, spine, throat and scapulae.

***Grandmaster Khor's important points:***

- Raise your head upwards through the *Bai Hui* acupoint
- Keep shoulders balanced, the spine straight and the pelvis level.
- Your knees should be over your feet, and your feet should be shoulder width apart.

## *Chi* meditation for the Microcosmic Orbit

We are going to start our *Chi* meditation by working on the main, vital energy circuit of the body. This is the circuit formed by the connection of the *Du Mai* (Governing Vessel) and *Ren Mai* (Conception Vessel). This is the Microcosmic Orbit. It concentrates on the torso and the head.

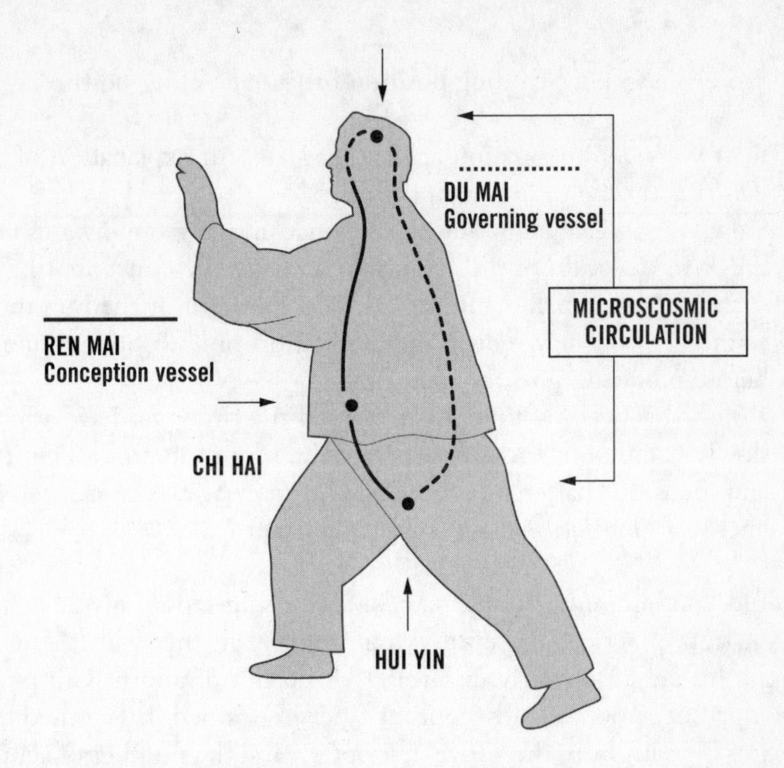


There are two ways in which *Chi* energy can be 'encouraged' to flow within this circuit. The first is by mentally focusing on acupoints on the *Du Mai* and *Ren Mai* meridians in sequence. The second is to imagine a small gold-coloured sphere of energy, about the size of a golf ball, travelling along the meridians passing each acupoint. It is also possible to combine these techniques. (A table listing the acupoints and their position on the body follows.)

When you first start the meditation, you may find your concentration is limited. Do not worry about this. Even if you succeed only in focusing on one point in early sessions, you are making progress. The first time you visualise each acupoint, you should try to maintain the visualisation of the energy sphere at the acupoint location, about one inch inside the body, for about five minutes. Be very aware of any physical changes, such as warmth, that you may feel in the area.

Do not be concerned if you feel the urge to wriggle or jerk, this is quite normal when energy blockages are dispersed. Any such symptoms should gradually diminish over time. If you have difficulty holding a visualisation, you can start off by placing your fingertips over the first few acupoints being visualised. (This becomes impossible later on, unless you are a contortionist!)

From the Quiet Standing position or Quiet Sitting posture:

- Start your *Chi* meditation at the *Tan Tien*. (An explanation of the *Tan Tien* can be found in Appendix 5.)
- Slowly open each acupoint in sequence, moving downwards along the *Ren Mai* and upwards along the *Du Mai*, by concentrating on each acupoint for five minutes. (Once you have opened up the acupoints, you may reduce the meditation time to one minute before proceeding to the next point.)
- When you become tired, or have used the time you have available, slowly bring your focus back along the meridians to the *Tan Tien* and focus on that area for a minute or two. Always re-centre your energy at *Tan Tien*—this is most important.

Should you encounter unpleasant or disturbing sensations during your meditation practice, re-centre your energy at the *Tan Tien*. If the symptoms are particularly disturbing, or do not diminish with practice, cease practice and seek advice from a person trained in *Chi* meditation.

It is obvious from the above description and the number of acupoints to be opened up in the Microcosmic Orbit that it is probably going to take six or more meditation sessions to open up all the acupoints. Do not be in any hurry.

***Grandmaster Khor's important points:***

- When moving the point of awareness, or the visualisation of the sphere, this should be done slowly and evenly. Imagine a ping-pong ball either slowly sinking or floating up through honey and you will have the correct imagery.
- Each time you have either opened up or focused on an acupoint, move the sphere along the meridian to the next point or return it to the *Tan Tien* to re-centre.

It is impracticable to focus on all the points located on the Governing (*Du Mai*) and Conception (*Ren Mai*) vessels. There are 52 of them. Thus, for this module, the points with major impact on the body's energy flows have been selected (see next page). Also, the movement of the point of visualisation through these selected points will effectively open up all of the remaining points on these meridians.

Remember to re-centre your energy.

**Acupoints on which to meditate in the Microcosmic Orbit**

| | |
|---|---|
| *Shenque* | Immediately behind the navel |
| *Chi Hai* | Three finger widths below the navel |
| *Guan Yuan* | Two finger widths above the pubic bone |
| *Qugu* | At the upper border of the pubic bone |
| *Hui Yin* | In the centre of the perineum (between the anus and the genitals) |
| *Yao Shu* | One inch up from the tip of the coccyx (tail bone), in the hiatus of the sacrum |
| *Ming Men* | Between the first and second lumbar vertebrae |
| *Zi Zhong* | Between the 11th and 12th thoracic vertebrae |
| *Feng Fu* | At the base of the skull |
| *Bai Hui* | At the midpoint of the line connecting the apex of the ears |
| *Yin Tang* | The midpoint between the eyebrows |
| *Su Liao* | At the tip of the nose |
| *Tian Tu* | In the notch of the bones at the base of throat (technically the centre of the suprasternal fossa) |
| *Shan Zhong* | In males, this is located between the nipples. In women, this is about an inch and a half from the base of the sternum, technically on a level with the fourth intercostal space |
| *Zhong Wan* | Four finger widths above the umbilicus |

## *Chi* meditation for the Macrocosmic Orbit

When you are comfortable with the Microcosmic Orbit, you can then proceed to open up the Macrocosmic Orbit. Whereas the Microcosmic Orbit involves only the torso and head, the Macrocosmic Orbit involves all of the limbs as well. In the Macrocosmic Orbit, you can either meditate on the points in both legs or arms at the same time, or treat each limb separately, one after the other.

**Acupoints on which to meditate in the Macrocosmic Orbit**

| | |
|---|---|
| *Shenque* | Immediately behind the navel |
| *Hui Yin* | In the centre of the perineum (between the anus and the genitals) |
| *Wei Zhong* | At the centre of the back of the knees |
| *Yong Quan* | At the soles of feet, in the junction of the anterior/middle sole |
| *Yin Bai* | On the big toe, just below the bottom of the toe-nail root |
| *Da Du* | Extends along the inside edge of the foot to the joint of the lower bone of the toe |
| *He Dig* | Top of the knee |
| *Hui Yin* | In the centre of the perineum (between the anus and the genitals) |
| *Ming Men* | Between the first and second lumbar vertebrae |
| *Da Zhi* | Between the spinous process of the seventh cervical vertebra and the first thoracic vertebra |
| *Qu Chi* | On the outside end of the elbow crease when the arm is flexed |

| | |
|---|---|
| *Lao Gong* | Centre of the palm |
| *Wai Guan* | Back of wrist, three finger widths from the crease |
| *Da Zhi* | Between the spinous process of the seventh cervical vertebra and the first thoracic vertebra |
| *Bai Hui* | A the midpoint of the line connecting the apex of the ears |
| *Shan Zhong* | In males, this is located between the nipples. In women, it is about an inch and a half from the base of the sternum, technically on a level with the fourth intercostal space |
| Shenque | Immediately behind the navel |

## Technique 2 Golden cloud meditation

This is a simple but effective meditation that uses diaphragmatic breathing and either the Quiet Standing or Quiet Sitting posture.

- Close your eyes and visualise yourself surrounded by a golden glowing cloud. As you breathe in, you can sense yourself drawing part of this glowing cloud inwards through your nose, down your throat and into your lungs. As you breathe in the golden glowing cloud, it warms the lining of your nose, breathing passageways and lungs. This is soft energising warmth and you can almost feel how healthy it is as it starts to spread further and further through your body with each in-breath. The lining of your nose, airways and lungs themselves begin to take on a golden glow and this glow begins to spread outwards into your body cavity with each in-breath. Once your whole torso is glowing, with each in-breath begin to draw the energy into your head, then your arms and hands and finally into your legs and feet.

- Continue until you visualise the whole of your body being warm, golden, glowing and energised. This cloud permeates you—not just your physical body but your mind, your emotions and your spirit. You are alive and energised but also peaceful and tranquil. If you have any problems of the body, the mind, the emotions or the spirit, feel the golden glowing energy healing you, repairing your body, making you tranquil and serene, dissolving any worry or fear, and brightening and uplifting your spirit until you feel vital and alive.

- Become secure in the knowledge that the golden glowing cloud is always present and it only has to be summoned by your mind. It will be there if you get tired or depressed, if you feel pain or need to be healed. Hold this thought in your mind as you half open your eyes. Maintain your breath and imagine the cloud still out there. You can almost see it underlying the air you breathe, the ground beneath you, and the physical objects that surround you. Then open your eyes fully, knowing that this is a meditation which never ends and that the golden glowing cloud is always present and available.

## Technique 3 Colour meditation

Like the golden cloud in the previous technique, when you meditate on colours, the colours should all have an energetic nature of being pure and glowing. They should be vibrant within themselves. The Chinese theory of the five elemental energy phases tells us that each organ system has a particular energy level or phase. Light has these same phases, which we perceive as different colours. Where the five-element phase of a colour is the same as an organ system, that phase or vibration is beneficial to the organ system in question.

If you have a problem with any part of the body, you can determine which organ system that it is related to and visualise that part of the body being filled with the vibrant associated colour.

As with the previous technique, you should use diaphragmatic breathing and either the Quiet Standing or Quiet Sitting posture.

| BODY AREA OR PART | ORGAN SYSTEM | MEDITATION COLOUR |
|---|---|---|
| Stomach, spleen, pancreas, blood | Stomach, spleen | Golden yellow |
| Liver, gall bladder, endocrine organs, bone, tendon, muscle | Liver, gallbladder | Spring green |
| Heart, pericardium, aorta, coronary and major arteries, sexual functions, nervous system, saliva, gastric juice, cerebrospinal fluid | Heart, small intestine | Ember red |
| Lung, rectum, colon, bronchiole, trachea, skin, sweat, urine | Lung, colon | Lustrous white |
| Kidney, bladder, urethra, ureter, adrenal gland, endocrine glands, sexual organs (testes or ovaries) | Kidney, bladder | Ocean blue |

## Technique 4 Sound meditation

We are all aware that sounds can have very distinct effects on our moods, emotions and energy. We have probably all heard that plants grow better when exposed to certain types of music (this should be treated with caution when applied to human beings—what is good for plants, such as manure in their diet, is not automatically recommended for us!).

The certain thing is that sound, as energy, will have an effect on us. After all, we do not just hear sound with our ears. The vibration or pressure waves that we perceive as sound affect every cell in our body. The sound that affects us most may well be our own voice.

It is our body that generates these pressure waves and the emotion that is carried on the voice is actually the emotional energy carried in the voice. Singing and chanting have long been used to change our emotional and spiritual state, our good moods. On the other hand, harsh, cruel, angry, bitter, hate-filled voices not only have a psychological impact, but there may be a direct physiological response as well. So it it easy to see that the voice can be a two-edged sword—it can heal or hurt others as well as ourselves.

In preform the sound mediation, you should use diaphragmatic breathing and either be in the Quiet Standing position or Quiet Sitting Posture.

- Concentrate on the sound you have chosen.
- As you breathe in, draw the sound into your body. Let it wash through you and travel deep within you.
- As you breathe out, allow the sound to travel out of your body.
- Continue in this manner for the time you have allowed to do the sound meditation.

## Technique 5 Bone breathing meditation

This is a very powerful technique. The ancient Chinese felt that the bones lay at the heart of our energy and strength (and indeed they are a major source of our blood). To strengthen themselves, the warrior priests would visualise themselves breathing energy into their bones.

To perform a bone breathing meditation, you should use diaphragmatic breathing and either the Quiet Standing or Quiet Sitting posture. Draw the energy into your bones on your in-breath, concentrating the energy of the bone on your out-breath. Unless you have a specific problem with a particular bone, focus on:

- The bones of your hands as a group
- The bones of your arms as a group
- Your spine
- The bones of your legs as a group
- The bones of your feet as a group.

## Technique 6 Positive Thinking

The power of positive thinking should not be underestimated in its ability to develop beneficial outcomes. It is not recommended that you dispense with more traditional medical approaches but rather that you supplement these treatments with positive thinking.

When using positive thinking, always remember that it is the power of the image that you hold in your mind that is important. You should not think about the sickness you want to overcome or it will be the image of sickness that you hold in your mind. Rather, the image should be of health and energy, particularly as these relate to the lungs or activities that involve the use of the lungs. The time immediately following your exercise session is great for some positive imagery.

## Technique 7 Smiling

The fact that the body and the mind are simply two sides of the same coin cannot be overstated. The smile is a great example of this. When our mental state is happy and vital, we smile. We don't have to think about it, we just do it. But, when we smile, the other side of the coin also comes into play. It has been shown that:

- the level of immunoglobins in the saliva increases, showing our immune system has kicked up a gear;
- the level of serotonin produced by the brain increases, making us more relaxed and less aware of pain'
- tension reduces within the muscles, other internal organs and body tissues;
- we move further in the direction of the relaxation response;
- we save energy because it takes less muscular effort to smile than it does to frown.

Part 4

# The FOF Program Acumassage Module

# The Acumassage Module

THE TRADITIONAL EASTERN APPROACH to acupressure and massage techniques—the combination of which I refer to as acumassage—differs from Western systems in both practice and theory. In the West, we tend to look at massage as something that is performed by a specialist when we have a medical problem—generally one that is related to the musculoskeletal system. In the East, while there are acumassage specialists available to deal with serious medical situations, the bulk of acumassage is performed within the family for the purpose of maintaining rather than restoring health.

Acumassage is a technique for maintaining a proper flow of *Chi* throughout the body. Because of the holistic nature of the body's energy flow, acumassage can be used to effect changes in areas of the body, far away from the area being massaged, but the techniques can also be used to treat a wide range of body ailments including physical, mental and emotional problems. The acumassage techniques included in the FOF Program have been selected on the basis that they can be used with minimal training, and can be applied either to yourself or someone else.

There are a number of techniques that will assist the effectiveness of the massage including:

- maintaining diaphragmatic breathing throughout the application of the technique;

- maintaining a relaxed upright posture wherever possible;
- understanding that it is not the amount of pressure that is important as much as the flow of *Chi* that you are using or stimulating;
- maintaining your focus on what you are doing throughout the application of the technique;
- remaining still and quiet for at least five minutes after performing the massage.

### HOW LONG AND OFTEN SHOULD YOU ACUMASSAGE?

Acumassage techniques can be applied over any length of time, but the best results will be obtained if the massage time, including quiet resting, exceeds 20 minutes. This allows biochemical as well as psychological relaxation.

There is no fixed requirement for how often you should acumassage each week, but about 20 minutes every couple of days is more than adequate from a health maintenance aspect.

### WHEN SHOULD YOU DO ACUMASSAGE?

This may be done just as effectively in the morning, afternoon or evening. Avoid times when you will be disturbed by interruptions.

### WHERE IS THE BEST PLACE TO DO ACUMASSAGE?

The location should be one where there is good circulation of air and no extreme environmental factors, such as heat or cold. Try not to perform acumassage in areas close to electrical equipment, such as computers and televisions, as these often produce positive ions and other pollutants from their components.

### SHOULD YOU USE MUSIC DURING ACUMASSAGE?

Appropriate music will aid in the relaxation response. The music should not contain a beat. Natural sounds such as birdsong, wind in the trees, ocean and stream sounds, can aid relaxation and soften any sudden unexpected sound. Do not use the radio and if you are using CDs and tapes, make sure that they last for the entire session.

### WHAT CLOTHING SHOULD YOU WEAR FOR ACUMASSAGE?

As long as clothing is loose and comfortable, it will suffice. Techniques can be applied over the surface of light clothing such as cotton t-shirts.

## ARE THERE ANY OTHER THINGS THAT CAN IMPROVE THE BENEFITS OF ACUMASSAGE ?

*Chi* energy is affected by the energy in the environment. It is therefore important that you pay attention to preparing an environment that supports the acumassage. For example, look at the eight environmental energies that are evaluated in Feng Shui:

| | |
|---|---|
| *Light* | The area should not have bright lights, particularly if they are in the field of vision of the subject. Obviously there must be enough light to carry out the massage safely. Colours should be subdued rather than garish. |
| *Sound* | Use an area that is not subject to sudden, loud or harsh sounds that may disturb the subject. |
| *Moisture* | The area should certainly not be damp but neither should it be too dry. Indoor waterfalls and fountains can be useful to moisten the air as well as provide soothing sound. |
| *Energy of form* | As far as possible, the physical objects in the massage area should be rounded or curved so that they offer no physical risk to people in the area. All materials and objects should be well maintained and there should be no clutter or untidiness. |
| *Energy of movement* | While the area should not feel still and stagnant neither should there be any strong flows of energy to which the subject is exposed. Make sure that the area is well ventilated with fresh air, but avoid exposure to draughts. |
| *Temperature* | The subject should be comfortably warm and not hot or cold. This will often depend on the ambient temperature, as well as the season. Do not expose people to direct flows of air from airconditioners but a slow fan, if necessary, may be used. |

| | |
|---|---|
| *Bio-energy* | In this, aquariums or plants can be helpful, but animal life, including birds, is too distracting. The negative ions produced by plants may also be useful. |
| *Aroma-energy* | The aroma should be both beneficial and pleasant. Lavender, for instance, relaxes, while pine and lemon can refresh and invigorate. |

**IMPORTANT POINTS ABOUT ACUMASSAGE**

- Remember to avoid force. Force makes the person receiving the treatment feel tense. Tension blocks the flow of *Chi*.
- Try to sense *Chi*. It is possible to feel the pulse of *Chi* at an acupoint, but this is quite different from your blood pulse. To feel the flow of *Chi* requires sensitivity and full awareness. Aim to obtain a strong, orderly regular pulsation.
- When working on acupoints, be aware of the condition of the tissue around the acupoint. This will tend to soften as the acupoint is opened up. Follow tension in as it releases, but do not press hard enough to create tension.
- If an acupoint is sensitive, use a slow circling of the fingers to loosen up the general area and only go deeper if the point becomes less tense and sensitive. If you are causing pain or discomfort, lighten pressure or abandon the point. All problems do not have to be fixed in one acumassage session.
- Be careful of long fingernails—this is acumassage not acupuncture! Remove jewellery that may present a hazard during massage.

## The FOF Program acumassage techniques

The acumassage techniques included in this module are:

- Technique 1 Abdominal massage
- Technique 2 Hand massage
- Technique 3 Ear massage
- Technique 4 Baojing ball massage

## Technique 1 Abdominal massage

This technique is very popular because of the general health benefits that occur when the acumassage is performed regularly. The movement tones the functioning of the digestive system and results in a feeling of vitality and ease.

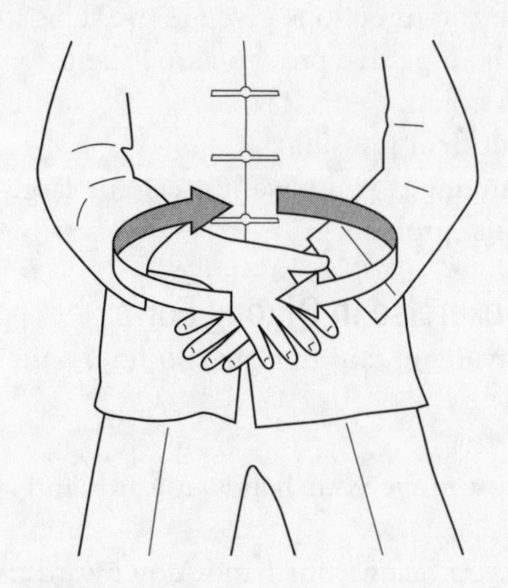

From the Quiet Standing position:

- Place the palm of your left hand on the abdomen so that your palm rests just inside the right pelvic bone. Place your right hand over your left. Keep your shoulders relaxed. The abdominal area remains covered during the movement but it will obviously be easier to perform the exercise in something like a t-shirt. The more layers of clothing you have and the more buttons, pockets and so forth that can get in the way, the more difficult it will be to perform this movement satisfactorily.
- Press down *gently* as you move your hands upwards to just under your rib cage. Still pressing gently, pull your hands across the top of the abdomen just under the rib cage. Push your hands downward along the left side of the abdomen to just inside the pelvic bone then pull them across to the right hip where you started.
- Repeat the circling of the abdominal area at least 36 times.
- Finish by bringing your hands to just under the navel as per Quite Standing position.

***Grandmaster Khor's important points:***

- Imagine that there is a beam of energy extending into the abdomen from your left palm that is moving and stirring the contents of the abdomen. While this is a physical massage, it is also a *Chi* massage and this means that the mental focus is much more important than the pressure applied.
- Always move in the directions given above. This follows the natural movement of the digestive process along the ascending, transverse and descending colon.
- Use a gentle but firm pressure.
- Avoid this technique if you have just eaten a large meal or are having abdominal problems.

### Performing this exercise in Qigong Form

Make sure you maintain an upright posture and synchronise your breathing as follows:

- Breathe in as you move your hands upwards and across to your left side.
- Breathe out as you bring your hands downwards and across to your right side.

WARNING

While this technique is generally quite safe, medical advice should be taken if the subject has had any recent surgery or if surgery is in prospect for conditions such as a growling appendix or bowel problems. This technique is also contraindicated for pregnancy. If there is any pain when performing this movement, lighten the pressure; if pain persists, cease the acumassage and seek medical advice before resuming the technique.

## Technique 2 Hand massage

The hand is related to the entire body. Therefore, working on the hand can be used as an overall health maintenance system. The hand is particularly useful for working on heart energy (centre of palm, and little and index finger), and this includes not only physical heart problems but emotional stress and tension. The hand area is also excellent for initiating the relaxation response.

From the Quiet Standing or Quiet Sitting position:

- Place your palms together. Rub your palms gently back and forward, interlocking fingers.
- Circle your palms over each other, making sure that you cover the whole of the palm, fingers and wrist crease.
- Roll over your right hand so that the palm of your left hand massages the back of all of your right hand. Roll back your right hand then roll over your left hand and repeat on your left hand.
- Take your left wrist and wrap your right thumb and fingers around it so that they meet, encircling your wrist at the wrist crease, and rotate the wrist backwards and forwards. Repeat for your right wrist.
- Use your right thumb to massage the area in the centre of the inside of your left arm, from the wrist crease to about four finger widths along the arm. Repeat with your left thumb on your right arm.
- Use your thumb and second finger to locate the *Nei Guan* (Pericardium 6) and *Wai Guan* (Triple Heater 5) points on your left forearm. Massage these by pressing your thumb and forefinger towards each other. Repeat on your right arm.
- Take your left hand in the tiger's mouth of your right hand, around the little finger edge of your left hand. Rub your right thumb back and forth from the crease of your left wrist to the base of the fingers. The underside of your right thumb should be in contact with the whole breadth of the left palm. Your right palm and the inside of your right fingers are simultaneously covering the whole back of your left hand and fingers. The tiger's mouth exerts pressure on the little finger of the left hand and the base of the little finger on the heart meridian. Repeat on your right hand.
- Emphasis can be changed to cover the centre of the palm, along the pericardium meridian and *Lao Gong*, and over the pad of the thumb and the wrist below it, covering the lung meridian.
- In a similar manner, use the tiger's mouth along the inside edge of the palm, between the junction of the thumb and fingers, with the emphasis over the *Hegu* point and along the back of the little finger.
- Take the thumb and fingers of your left hand one-by-one between the thumb and fingers of your right hand. Roll your right thumb

and fingers around each left digit, from the base to the tip. Press in slightly as your fingers pass the base of the nail leaving the digit with a slight flicking motion. Make sure that the pulling pressure applied is gentle. On no account should there be any excessive strain on any of the joints. Repeat on your right hand.

***Grandmaster Khor's important points:***

- Remain relaxed.
- Do not twist or pull forcefully on the finger joints.

## Technique 3 Ear massage

Many people are surprised that we spend time massaging the ear, believing that it is simply a flap of cartilage and skin designed to improve the focusing of sound waves. However, when we actually look at the anatomy of the ear, we find that it is very complex and has one of the body's most intricate systems of nerves and blood vessels.

The two ears have some 260 acupressure points. Another clue to the importance of the ears is the universal liking, not only by people but by cats, dogs and other mammals, for having them stroked and rubbed. In fact, just as other areas of the body, such as the hands, feet and abdomen, have energetic effects on the entire body so does the ear.

### DRAGON NIBBLES THE EARS

This massage exercise is particularly good for improving blood and energy circulation in the limbs and is therefore beneficial to those who suffer from cold feet and hands or cramps within the limbs. Because of the increase in blood circulation, it is also good for joint problems within the limbs. When massaging someone else:

- Start with your thumbs on the outside of the tops of the ears, with your index and middle fingers at the back of the ears so that the rims are gently pressed between your thumbs and fingers.
- Gently circle your thumbs and first fingers so that the rims of the ears are both slightly pulled and stretched and gently pressed. As the top of the circle is reached, slide your thumbs and fingers down

slightly so that gradually the whole rim of the ear is massaged and the thumbs and fingers finish at the tip of the earlobe. Then, without losing contact with the ears, slide your thumbs and fingers up along the rim to the starting position.

- Repeat the movement, from the top of the ear to the earlobe and then sliding back, 12 times. Each massaging circle should be done to the count of two. You should feel the ear becoming warm, full and flexible.

For self-massage, use the following variations:

- Work on one ear at a time, which allows the head to be tilted and thus avoid stress in the shoulder.
- Place your thumb behind the top of the rim of your ear and your index finger on the top of the front of the rim, and follow the instructions set out above.

***Grandmaster Khor's important points:***

- Focus your attention on the area between your thumb and index finger.
- Be very careful of ear jewellery and do not massage over the jewellery or get your hands caught up in it.

## EARLOBE MASSAGE

As well as having benefits similar to the previous exercise, massaging the earlobes is an overall health tonic because, in Taoist traditions, the earlobes are associated with longevity. This is related to the location of the hypothalamus, pineal and pituitary glands within the head, and massaging of the earlobes stimulates the functioning of these glands and affects the endocrine system. When doing this massage on someone else:

- With your thumbs over the front of the earlobe and your index finger at the back of the earlobe, gently press and pull the earlobes downwards and outwards.
- The pulling separating movement should be done to the count of six, and repeated 10 to 12 times.

For self-massage, use the following variation:

- Place your thumb behind your earlobes and your index finger on the front of the earlobe, and follow the technique instructions.

***Grandmaster Khor's important points:***

- Focus your attention on the earlobe.
- Do not press on ear jewellery.

## EAR STROKING MASSAGE

This massage exercise stimulates the inner part of the outer ear known as the cymba conchae and cavum conchae. These areas of the ear are associated with the body's internal organs.

Follow these steps to perform this ear massage on someone else:

- Using the thumb side of your first finger, make short striking motions up and down between the back of the ears and where the ears connect to the skull (around the area of the mastoid bone). The movement should be quick but not overly vigorous on the head, as this will create resistance and discomfort in the subject's neck muscles.
- These striking motions are about 3–4 centimetres apart. Each motion is slightly lower than the last so that the whole back area of the ear, from the top to the base, is included. The main point of contact should be the first and second segments of your index finger along the connection of the ears to the scalp.
- When you reach the base of the ear, slide your finger back to the starting position and move down the ear again with short vigorous striking motions. This entire movement should be repeated at least six times.

For self-massage, use the following variation:

- Massage one ear at a time, tilting your head in that direction, to cause less stress on your shoulders.
- The striking motion is upward and should start at the base of ear.

***Grandmaster Khor's important points:***

- Focus your attention on the area between the ear and the skull.
- Be careful of ear jewellery.
- Beware of sharp fingernails.

## Technique 4 Baojing ball massage

Baojing balls, sometimes called *Yin–Yang* balls or Chinese health balls, are small balls, usually made of silver or enamel, that are used to maintain the health of the hands.

Generally two balls are held in the hand and rotated around each other. The idea is to ensure that the balls do not clack together—as they move around each other, they can remain either constantly in contact or, in a more advanced movement, constantly apart.

The Baojing balls are quite weighty, and this allows them to stimulate the acupoints and reflexology zones over which they pass while at the same time toning the muscles in the hands and arms.

There are many benefits of using Baojing balls, including:

- The pressure of smooth objects over the palm tends to initiate the relaxation response, thus reducing stress and tension and engaging the 'healing and growth mode' of the body.
- A number of important acupoints are simulated, particularly *Lao Gong*.
- The rhythmic flexing of the muscles and tendons required to keep the balls circling stimulates all six of the organ meridians in the hands. Also, when you keep the balls circling apart, you use the pads of your fingertips and this encourages both the release of excess energy and the flow of *Chi* energy between meridians.
- All the hand joints are well exercised but not in a strenuous manner. This is especially beneficial to those with arthritic conditions.
- As noted above, the muscles in the arms become toned through supporting the weight of the balls, and this also increases the flow of blood and *Chi* through the arms.

### WHAT SIZE BAOJING BALLS SHOULD YOU USE?

Baojing balls are found in several sizes, as are people's palms! You should start off with the largest size with which you are comfortable. Remember that your ability to manage Baojing balls will increase rapidly but, in general terms, the larger the Baojing balls the greater the benefits available.

It's interesting to note that some experienced Chinese are adept at keeping four Baojing balls circling separately in each palm, even though Chinese people in general are not noted for having large hands.

### WHAT TYPE OF BAOJING BALLS SHOULD YOU USE?

Baojing balls are made of various materials such as metal coated, enamel coated, and cloisonné. There are also some health balls with various bumps and knobs available. In general, the smoother the balls the better the relaxation response. The rougher or more irregular the balls, the more stimulation of *Chi* and acupoints.

Metal-coated Baojing balls may not look as pretty as enamel or cloisonné, but the balls will better survive being dropped (as they will be!). There is some comment that metal Baojing balls are better at retaining the *Chi* of the user but I know of no research about this.

### WHY DO BAOJING BALLS MAKE A SOUND?

Baojing balls are designed to make sounds with *Yin* and *Yang* natures. Sound is vibration, so each set of balls is vibrating with a *Yin* and *Yang* tone. This can help balance the energy of the body, both in transmission of energy through the palm and the actual hearing of the sound.

### ARTHRITIS AND EXERCISING WITH BAOJING BALLS

The use of Baojing balls can be particularly useful for arthritis sufferers. Not only does the use of these balls increase flexibility of joints, but they gently tone the muscles and have positive calming and *Chi* stimulation effects that can influence the health of the whole body.

I have seen students suffering from arthritis who, when they started Baojing ball exercises, could do no more than hold one ball in the palm of their hand and open and close their fingers. Gradually they became able to turn the ball in their palm, then they were able to add the second ball, and finally to rotate the two balls. This greatly increased their overall flexibility for other daily tasks and reduced pain and stiffness within the hand joints.

## BAOJING BALL EXERCISES

Each person will have a different degree of flexibility in the hands. Some people may have initial difficulty just supporting and moving the balls in the hand. Others will have greater flexibility. Practice the following exercise to the level with which you are comfortable.

- Start by being comfortable holding only one Baojing ball in your hand. You should be able to turn your hand upwards and downwards, and wrap and unwrap your fingers around the ball.

- Repeat using two Baojing balls.
- Start to move the balls around each other in the palm of your hand in a circling motion but don't worry if they clack together at first.
- Practice and eliminate clacking by keeping the balls smoothly together.
- Circle the balls around in the palm of your hand without the balls touching. Gradually get the balls circling further and further apart until they are riding over the base and first segments of your fingers.
- Repeat the exercise but reverse the direction of the circling.

***Grandmaster Khor's important points:***

- Remember that you should spend equal amounts of time exercising the left and the right hand.
- If you want to save time, you can have a set of Baojing balls in each hand simultaneously.
- Don't practice over stone floors and don't practice with bare feet. Dropped baojing balls don't survive the first instance, and your feet won't survive the second! A Baojing ball dropped from on an exposed toe can literally leave a lasting impression!
- The exercise is most effective, and comfortable, when your shoulders, elbows and wrist joints are kept relaxed. It helps to reduce stress tensions stored in these areas.
- Keeping the balls moving without clacking requires constant, focused attention. In a sense, this is a type of meditation and it can increase your ability to concentrate and focus while at the same time initiating the relaxation response.

## Technique 5 Moxabustion

Moxabustion is the process of burning herbs close to the body. It has been found to be a most effective way of getting heat into the body and it can also be used to warm the joints with other positive benefits.

Through this technique, the *Chi* energy of the herb is transferred into the body's energy meridian system. It is interesting to note that studies have shown that the tissue around an acupoint builds up to a higher temperature when moxa herbs are being burned than when other heat sources of the same temperature are placed the same distance away.

The simplest way to apply moxabustion is in the form of a moxa stick. Moxa sticks are available from most Chinese herb shops.

WARNING
While the following technique is generally quite safe, avoid use without medical advice on persons with acute conditions of high blood pressure or if pregnant. Do not use this technique when climatic conditions are hot. If there is any giddiness, nausea, pain or other adverse signs, immediately discontinue the technique.

## MOXA VITALITY EXERCISE

This technique is particularly good for energising the body in the winter months. In a sitting position:

- Light the end of the moxa stick and direct the burning end of the stick towards the *Hegu* point (in the fleshy tissue between the thumb and index finger).
- Keep the end of the moxa stick about 3–4 centimetres from the *Hegu* point, moving the moxa stick away and towards the point in slow motions. The area will feel warm and the texture of the skin will become oily. Continue for 3–5 minutes on the *Hegu* point of each hand.

***Grandmaster Khor's important points:***
- Remain focused or you will end up stabbing yourself with the hot end of the moxa stick.
- The inwards motion should be aimed at generating as much heat as you can comfortably tolerate. You should not proceed to the point where there is any pain.
- Do not use moxa herbs on any area where there is injury, skin problems or swelling of the tissue in the *Hegu* area.
- Most important, the *Hegu* point should not be used when pregnant.
- Discontinue if you experience negative sensations before or after moxa treatment.

Part 5

# The FOF Program *Chi* Nutrition/Environment Module

# The *Chi* Nutrition/ Environment Module

THE MODERN WORLD tends to carry it's 'No pain, no gain' philosophy into diet and we commonly get the idea that eating is about deprivation and denial and that foods are good for us if they taste bad. Nothing could be further from the truth. While food is regarded as the first line of defence for the body, it must also nourish the emotions and spirit.

When we look at the Chinese diet, we see one of the world's great cuisines—it focuses on taste, aroma, texture, colour and presentation. This does not mean that *Chi* nutrition requires you to eat Chinese-style food—these principles can be applied to any style of diet. Anyone can enjoy eating their food while also providing the body, mind and spirit with what it needs.

## A *Chi* nutrition approach to diet

The standard approach to nutrition is to look at the food you buy and eat (ingest to be technical) but in fact, what is important to us is the food that is actually assimilated through the digestive system into the blood as macronutrients or micronutrients. (Macronutrients include proteins, fats and carbohydrates, while micronutrients include vitamins and minerals.)

In traditional Chinese approaches, there is much less distinction between the daily eating of food and the application of preventative and corrective health regimes than in the West. In the Chinese approach, food is taken to maintain a correct individual energy balance and is thus primarily preventative in nature, although it has a major secondary role as an energy balance cure. When one's sense of well-being is not what it should be, or when sickness strikes, the first inclination of the Chinese is to look at modifying the diet and there are many 'food cures' in China, both in traditional approaches and in modern health practices.

The factors that affect the quantity and quality of food nutrients that make it to your bloodstream include:

- the freshness of the food when it is eaten;
- the methods used to store the food before and after purchase;
- the way the food is cooked;
- how the food is combined in a meal and its presentation;
- the temperature of the food when it is eaten;
- the environment in which the food is eaten;
- the emotional state in which the food is eaten.

In addition, the quantity and quality of energy (*Chi*) within food itself, and how this is affected by the above factors, must be taken into account.

*Chi* nutrition recognises that everyone has individual nutrition requirements so it incorporates techniques and approaches that will meet your needs while providing you with an enjoyable diet.

## Factor 1 Assessing and selecting food

This technique involves maximising the quantity of the *Chi* in the actual food at the point of purchase or collection.

### The importance of selecting food

When people evolved as hunter–gatherers, they did not have to worry about how the food that they had hunted or gathered had grown and developed, since each plant and animal had developed in its own natural way. Rather, the problem was finding and catching the food on a regular enough basis to satisfy the needs of the family group.

The introduction of agriculture and the domestication of animals largely solved the food quantity problems faced by the hunter–gatherer societies. However, as it commonly happens, the result was a trade-off.

When people started to produce their own food, the negative aspects of the trade-off were:

- Reduction in the variety of the diet—only plants that could be easily grown or animals that could be easily domesticated would form part of the new diet.
- Decrease in quality of the diet—the growing of foods in unnatural locations and the keeping of animals in unnatural lifestyles impacts on the quantity of the *Chi* that could be obtained from the food.

The nature of the *Chi* of any animal or plant changes if there is a dramatic change in the environment, diet and physical structure of the animal or plant. Any change in the taste of the food can be taken as an indication of such an energy change. (This deterioration of quality has only increased as technology and food production methods have advanced, for example with hormones and antibiotics being added to the food to increase the efficiency of its production.) It should also be emphasised that, whilst the trade-off had negative effects, it still represented a great leap forward for most of humanity because:

- length of life increased;
- human societies grew larger and more complex;
- there was increased opportunity for mental, physical and spiritual development.

It is also true that some hunter–gatherer societies of great cultural and human significance, such as the Australian Aborigines, have been severely damaged by exposure to modern industrial societies, but this damage does not seem to relate primarily to food consumption pattern changes.

Whatever we think of the various agricultural and industrial revolutions our species has undergone, it is how we deal with the negative effects of those revolutions that affects our lives. The following suggestions aim to improve the quantity of the *Chi* in the foods in our diet. Note, if you can satisfy all these requirements you are doing very well.

## Choosing fruits and plants

Wherever possible, choose fruits and plants in the following order of preference:

| | |
|---|---|
| *Organically grown* | That is, grown without pesticides and artificially produced chemical stimulants. |
| *In season* | There two main reasons for this: Firstly, the nature of the *Chi* is appropriate; and secondly, there has been less opportunity for deterioration and the use of artificial preservative processes. (Sun-drying for preservation and storage in dry, dark, cool locations can sometimes improve the *Chi* of certain foods.) |
| *Healthy-looking* | For healthy, read natural; and not the artificially enhanced colours that are often found, for instance, in apples and egg yolks. |
| *Locally grown* | If grown locally (and in season) then the nature of the *Chi* associated with the food should be 'in tune' with the *Chi* of the local environment and is more likely to meet the body's needs. If foods are not grown locally, select foods from an environment where the seasons are the same as the local area. |

## Choosing meats, poultry and fish

Wherever possible, choose meats, poultry and fish in this order:

- Animals raised in their natural environment, rather than in closed environments, such as batteries.
- Domesticated animals that have lived a life and had a diet as close as possible to the animal's natural environment. They should also be organically raised and free of hormones and antibiotics, for example free-range chickens. Avoid fish, fowl and meat products produced on an intensive farming basis.
- Healthy-looking animals—read natural and not the artificially enhanced colours that are often found, for instance, in meats laced with MSG (monosodium gluten).
- Animals raised locally (and in season). The nature of *Chi* associated with the food should be 'in tune' with the *Chi* of the local environment and is more likely to meet the body's needs. If foods are not grown locally, select foods from an environment with seasons the same as the local area.

## Factor 2 Storing, transporting and preserving food

This technique involves maintaining, enhancing or improving the nature and quantity of the *Chi* in the food during any storage or preservative process that takes place between the time of acquisition and the time of consumption. In this technique, we consider the effect on the nature and quality of *Chi* that may occur from the:

- manner in which food items were harvested, transported and stored;
- length of time between harvesting and consumption of food;
- methods used to preserve the food during the time between harvesting and consumption.

In most cases, we will not know the manner in which the food item has been harvested, transported or stored and we have to rely on the appearance of the food to tell us what it has been subjected to. Look for signs of bruising, loss of colour, excessive dryness or moistness of the food.

If you are harvesting, transporting or storing the food yourself, try to avoid carrying out any of these processes in excessive heat or dampness, as these accelerate the degenerative effect. The obvious exceptions are naturally moist foods, which should be kept moist (preferably in a sealed environment where moisture will not be lost). The food should be subjected to as little physical damage as possible.

In most cases, foods should be stored in cool, dry, dark areas. Again, this obviously excludes moist foods, which should not be allowed to dehydrate, and the best solution is to seal them in environments where this will not happen.

As can be seen from the above, it is virtually impossible to talk about the transportation and storage of food without bringing up the process of preservation.

There are many methods of preserving foods, from non-invasive storage in a cool, dry place to the full gamut of chemical preservation and radiation. Some of these are sun-drying, smoking, salting, pickling, sealing, freezing, irradiating, and chemically preserving. Each preservative process has a specific effect on the quantity and nature of the *Chi* inside the food. However, such effects are not always destructive of the *Chi* quantity. For instance:

- Sun-drying, dehydration and smoking can concentrate the *Chi* energy of a food.
- Pickling and salting can change the nature of the *Chi*—this can be good or bad depending on individual needs and on what you want the nature of the *Chi* to be.
- Freezing seems, at best, a neutral process that can slow down the loss of *Chi*.
- Chemical preservatives should not be opposed simply because they are artificial, but because they usually introduce an unknown factor in terms of how they will affect *Chi*. Any substance ingested can have the ability to affect the body's *Chi*.
- The jury is still out on irradiation. It is not an additive and one must be suspicious that some of the current responses are not simply emotional in nature, coming from people who would probably have opposed the discovery of fire if they had been around at the time!

An old Chinese adage warns that you should not eat something unless it can rot but you should not eat it when it does rot. The basic point here is that if a food does not rot, either its *Chi* structure is so stable that living organisms cannot absorb it, or it is so 'unhealthy' no other organism will touch it. Either way, it is not likely to do the human organism much good! To a certain extent, preserving processes help to solve this age-old problem.

With the exception of some foods which have undergone natural preservation processes that actually enhance the *Chi*, such as pickling and fermentation, the fresher the food, the better it is for you. So, in general, buy small amounts of fresh food frequently, rather than large amounts that need to be stored.

## Factor 3 Preparing food

This technique involves maintaining, enhancing or changing the nature and quantity of the *Chi* in the food during the preparation process, in relation to cooking, meal design and presentation.

This technique is basically about the total creation of a meal, beginning with its preparation. While in the West we tend to look at the overall diet, we can often ignore the importance of the meal in its own right. Yet, it is in the total creation of the meal that many important factors come into play.

For example, the Chinese believe that food should have the following qualities, and be:

- pleasing in aroma;
- pleasing to the eyes;
- pleasing in taste;
- pleasing to the body.

These factors can only be considered at the meal level, and not for the overall diet. However, first we have to ask:

- Why do these qualities matter? Isn't healthy food healthy regardless of how it looks or smells?
- How can we ensure that the food in a meal has these qualities, especially if these qualities are not natural to the food or if we have specific dietary needs?

No one would deny that having an argument in the middle of a meal, or worrying during a meal, affects its benefits. Such things are known to have a dramatic impact on the digestive process, and on the ability to produce the required digestive juices. The Chinese take this one step further—they believe that the more the senses are pleasantly stimulated, the more we will focus favourable impressions on the meal and so the more effective will be the absorption of *Chi* into the body. If the food is unattractive, then our focus on the food will be negative and this will interfere with the absorption of *Chi*.

However, while in general a diet must be balanced, there is no reason why every individual meal must be balanced. In fact, since our body's digestive system must cope with different foods in different ways, which are often opposed, the concept of having a little bit of everything at each meal is a most unhealthy one.

Limiting the number of food types does not mean we have to limit the number of food tastes. For example, instead of having three dinners on consecutive days each meal made up of one type of meat, one type of green vegetable and a source of carbohydrate, it would be much better to have one meal of mixed meats, one meal of mixed vegetables and then one meal of mixed carbohydrates. The overall dietary intake is exactly the same, but the digestive problems are reduced and the possibility of making each meal quite different from the preceding one is enhanced.

At any individual meal, it is possible to add supplementary foods as long as they are consumed in a quantity and manner that does not adversely affect the overall balanced diet. Such supplementary foods can also be balanced so that they have opposite effects, which are then neutral in total effect on your energy balance.

There are many techniques of cooking, preparing and presenting food and all of these will influence both the quantity and nature of the *Chi*. Some combinations of food energies are beneficial, whilst others are deleterious. The proportions of foods should not be ignored, and neither should the effect of various spices, salts, sauces and herbs.

## Factor 4 Cooking

The discovery of fire led to the possibility of 'cooking' food. This was a major advance in humanity. Cai Jinfeng, put it succinctly in his book, *Eating Your Way to Health*:

> Cooked food is not only tasty but also greatly lessens the chance of contracting disease, especially those through the digestive tract. Cooked food strengthens the body's resistance to disease, since the nutrients in the food, especially the proteins, are more readily digested and absorbed.

'Cooking' is now so important in the total 'preparing' of food that the two terms have come to virtually mean the same thing—with cooks now preparing our salads! In this book, however, we shall preserve the distinction and the terms 'to cook' or 'cooking' will refer to the preparation of food involving the application of heat.

The art of cooking provides some of the best evidence that there is 'something' (*Chi*) involved that makes it more than simple chemistry. Who would want to eat a meal prepared by someone who thinks that there is no difference between cooking and chemistry, and that cooking is only the transfer of thermal heat energy into a food substance to provoke certain chemical reactions? (Unfortunately, it's easy to suspect that this concept is applied all too frequently by the technologists who design and prepare much of the pre-processed food we eat today!)

The process of cooking is so much more than the amount of thermal energy absorbed by a food over a given period of time. One food, depending on how heat is applied, can have myriad effects, depending on how it is treated: whether it is cooked over an open flame, gas, electricity, charcoal, and so on; the distance between the food and the heat source; the nature and shape of any materials between the food and the heat source, such as a griddle, hotplate or saucepan, and the utensils used; and the nature of movement that the food undergoes while in the presence of the heat source.

Another advantage associated with cooking is that it offers the opportunity to eat the food at a temperature that matches the body's temperature. There is little advantage, and considerable danger, in ingesting food that is at higher than body temperature. While on the other hand, many of the chemical processes of digestion are impaired by lower temperatures. When food is delivered at lower than body temperatures, digestion slows until the food has been heated up. This means that the peristalsis may have already taken the food into areas not designed to receive partially digested food. It also means that heat will flow from the core of the body to the stomach. Lowering of core body temperature can interfere with metabolic functions and predispose the body to infection and illness.

The Chinese recognise that the stomach is designed to best carry out its digestive functions at body temperature. They also believe that the most beneficial method of eating is to eat a broth or soup at body temperature, particularly important where the body is in a weakened state from illness, injury or old age. (Interestingly, these are also the type of situations where soups and broths would be served in the West.)

Lin Yutang, a noted Chinese Philosopher, states:

> Chinese medicines are often served as stews and called soups. It is made like an ordinary soup, in that it must be made with the proper regard for the mixing of flavour and ingredients. The stew is designed not just to attack the illness but to nourish and strengthen the body as a whole.

AN ANCIENT CHINESE PROVERB ADVISES:

FIRST, DRINK SOUP WHEN EATING A MEAL,
SO THAT IN OLD AGE THE BODY
WILL NOT BE HARMED.

## Cooking and the nutritional values of food

An important issue is loss of nutritional value in food as a result of cooking. Bob Flaws, an expert in traditional Chinese medicine, uses the following example to deal with this problem. Flaws notes that the critical aspect of nutrition, in so far as the body is concerned, is not the nutritional value of the food ingested (taken into the digestive system) but the nutritional value assimilated into the body less the energy costs of such assimilation.

As an example of this, an item of food may have 100 nutritional units (NU) in its raw state but, due to its raw state, only 75 per cent of the NU might be digested (losing 25 NU) and the energy expended by the body in assimilating the food might use another 10 NU. As a result, the body has a net gain of 65 NU. That is:

100 NU (raw food) - 25 (lost in digestion) – 10 (energy expended)
= 65 NU gained

If the item of food is cooked, the total nutritional value might fall to 90 NU, but the amount absorbed in digestion might rise to 90 per cent (losing 9 units) and energy expended in digestion might fall to 5 NU. As a result, the net energy gain is 76 NUs. That is:

90 NU (cooked food) - 9 (lost in digestion) – 5 (energy expended)
= 76 NU gained

Thus, apart from other benefits of cooking, the net NU gain to the consumer may be actually increased through the cooking process, even though the number of NU in the food is reduced from its raw state.

# Factor 5 Meal design

It should be immediately realised that there is a great difference between meal design and diet design. There are many foods that should be a part of your diet that should not be present together in the one meal.

Eating starchy foods such as bread with high protein foods like meat is an example of a food combination the body will find difficult to digest properly. Apart from the loss of nutrition, improperly digested food may result in toxins being produced. Their energies are incompatible and so are the chemical reactions that may occur (or fail to occur) when these foods are eaten together. It is important, when reading any nutrition book, that you distinguish between general nutrition rules and guidelines and the conditions that must apply for a meal.

## Factor 6 Food presentation

In the East, the presentation and appearance of food is seen as being important to the overall meal. The art of food presentation is raised to extremely high aesthetic standards by the Japanese in a form they call 'Mukimono'. Paintings can be read as the artist's recreation of a *Chi* pattern, thus having the attributes of the original *Chi* pattern. This applies to any arrangement of a physical structure, be it a building, painting or garden, and, of course, the physical presentation of a meal also contains a *Chi* pattern.

Thus, the plate on which a meal is served, the physical layout of the food, the blending of colours, tastes and aromas and so on, all represent a multi-dimensional art form that is no less valuable for being transitory. In *The Art of Presenting Food*, Sallie Williams sums up the process:

> Each raw ingredient has its own meaning and the finished piece often represents a story. Like a Haiku poem (Japanese), the feeling meant to be elicited is often too subtle for the Western mind.

Presentation is important at every meal, be it a formal dinner, picnic or even a TV dinner. Presentation implies more than a pretty plate—it means the creation of a whole eating environment. If the participants at a meal are uncomfortable and disturbed, they will not benefit as they should from the meal. Look at temperature, ventilation, light, sound, comfort of seating, space, and so on. However, don't look at these things purely from the point of creating a bland environment in which none of these things are noticed—try to create an ambience.

It is not for nothing that restaurants incorporate log fires and artificial fountains in their décor, or that many restaurants have expensive views and locations. As a general rule, when a person is eating out, they will first look at the environment and decide if it is 'comfortable' for them to eat in. Only then will they look at menu and price.

## Factor 7 Eating

This technique involves maintaining or enhancing the quantity of *Chi* in the food through the food consumption process.

This process dovetails neatly with the previous techniques where the food has been carefully selected, prepared, designed and presented so that it will appeal to all the senses and enhance the quality of the *Chi*.

Now, the consumers must play their role. If you talk through magnificent music, or if you give a detailed picture a cursory glance, you would not expect to derive much benefit.

As a consumer of a meal, you have a similar responsibility to make sure that you get the best out of your meal. This should not be a burden, it should be a delight, but, like the creation or appreciation of any art, it requires an ability to focus on what one is doing. Also, the greater understanding you have of the art, the greater will be your enjoyment and benefit.

There are a number of factors to consider, including the environment in which we eat and the way in which we consume our food. In general, however, the *Chi* must be settled and the *shen* raised.

## Factor 8 Digestion

This technique involves maintaining or enhancing the quantity of *Chi* in the food through the digestion process. There are five 'areas' of digestion—mouth, stomach, duodenum, small intestine, and large intestine. We can assist the digestive process by doing the following:

- Allow time to eat;
- Be aware of food temperature;
- Chew food well, in order to aid saliva production as well as digestion;
- Be aware of emotions when eating, as stress responses inhibit production of digestion-aiding mucous;
- Gentle massaging exercises during the digestive process will aid peristalsis.

A meal is not over when the last mouthful has been ingested. In fact, the time immediately following a meal is critical, for this is the time when the structural *Chi* is broken down and released within the body.

While everyone appears to agree that vigorous exercise after a meal is not appropriate, there seems to be some variation of opinion as to whether one should rest or partake of mild exercise after a meal.

The proponents of rest will often point out that many animals do appear to rest after a meal. On closer inspection, however, such animals often turn out to be carnivores operating on the 'feast or famine' principle. That is, a carnivore never really knows where its next meal is coming from and will therefore gorge itself when it does secure a meal. This makes movement uncomfortable.

In the case of people, however, it is to be hoped that they will have adopted the principles outlined here, and also finished the meal when they are about 80 per cent replete. In this case, a gentle walk will serve to stimulate the circulatory and energy systems without over-exciting them. A walk in pleasant surroundings can also serve to place the body's energetic systems in a 'receptive' state, ideally suited to the digestion of energy as well as of physical food substances. This will aid in the proper digestion of the food.

## The Environment

The last, but definitely not least important, aspect of the FOF Program relates to our environment. This refers to the places where we live, eat and work and also the chemicals and energies that we come into contact with our bodies.

The higher the toxic load of our environments the more stress we put on our biological systems, including the immune system. We need to examine our environment and identify areas where we can reduce the toxic load.

### In our homes

Get rid of carcinogens that contain pesticides, fly sprays, cleaning products and so forth. The products we use to clean our teeth and hair often contain troubling chemicals. Read the product labels and avoid anything that contains sodium laurel sulphate (nearly all toothpastes do!) and propyl glycol. While the levels of these chemicals in these products would not increase the risk of disease, they certainly add to the overall toxic load on our bodies.

Treat any change in your environment with appropriate caution. If you buy a new home, furniture or home appliance be aware that many of these may release unpleasant and dangerous chemicals. This toxic load can be reduced by good ventilation, the use of an air ioniser and plenty of plants placed around the home.

## Our work environment

Modern offices have little ventilation and hundreds of positive-ion producers, such as computers. To avoid a highly toxic environment place plants around the office and on your desk or plug in an air ioniser. In air-conditioned environments drink plenty of fresh water—not coffee.

Be careful of the light you are exposed too. The light provided by fluorescent tubes creates the wrong wavelengths and may depress the immune system. If you cannot persuade your boss to put in full spectrum lighting (you might mention that these have been proved to raise productivity and reduce absenteeism) get a full spectrum lamp and put in on your desk.

## Our cars

An overlooked environment, in terms of toxic load, is our cars. Before we even start the engine, we need to think about all the cleaning agents used on the interior! Open the window and allow fresh air to flow through as much as possible. If the sun has raised the temperature inside the car to 40 degrees or more you may have a chemical soup stewing within the cabin. In this case it is best not to get straight into the car but rather open the doors and windows and allow fresh air to blow through before commencing your journey.

If your garage is part of your house rather than a separate building, leave your car on the driveway for 30 minutes or so before garaging it—the heat of the engine will continue to release volatile chemicals for about this period of time. Healthy houses have good flow-through ventilation but this ventilation works against you with a hot car. If your bedroom is above the garage this is particularly important. It is best to have non-porous flooring between you and your car.

## Be sensible

We can, of course, get quickly paranoid about radiation, carcinogens, electromagnetic fields and so forth to which we are exposed. The fact is that humans have been exposed to low levels of these throughout our evolution and the body has pretty effective coping mechanisms. What has really changed over the last few decades is the quantities and levels of the substances that we are exposed to. There is a good argument to be made for the fact that our bodies are suffering 'toxic overload'.

The logical thing to do is to seek to reduce this overload to a reasonable level, but without worrying ourselves sick that we cannot remove all of the chemical and energetic toxins from our environment.

## Appendix 1

# Healthy Relaxation

### What is relaxation?

RELAXATION IS A TERM that causes all sorts of problems because different people mean quite different things when they talk about it. To the average person, the type of image that springs to mind includes lying on a beach, reclining in a hammock, or some form of 'collapsed inactivity'. The last image we tend to summon up when thinking of relaxation is the image of ourselves engaged in physical exercise.

However, if you have ever had the misfortune to be confined to bed for an extended period, you will soon find out exactly what such inactivity does to your body and how stressed it soon becomes from such 'relaxing activity'! In fact, one of the worst forms of torture is to confine a person in a cramped area where they cannot stretch or move.

The reason why hospitals these days try to get patients up and about as soon as possible after surgery or illness is not due to the economic cost of keeping them in care, but because it is healthier for patients to be up and moving as soon as it is safe to do so. Prolonged inactivity leads to all sorts of complications, such as:

- faster, shallower breathing due to compression of lungs;
- weakened cardiovascular system due to deterioration of muscles;
- increased pressure on the heart because of inactivity in venous blood return system;
- under-performing immune system due to slower movement of lymph fluid;
- decalcification of the skeletal system (leading to osteoporosis) because of lack of weight-bearing exercise;
- increased risk of depression, which is statistically greater in those less active; and
- inability to properly maintain blood pressure.

It is important, however, that we do not to leap to the contrary and improper view that we should avoid lying down. Stress is reduced and we are in our most relaxed state when there is a proper overall balance between activity and rest. Hence, true relaxation is the continual search for a balance in activities and lifestyle that delivers optimum health.

To avoid confusion about what relaxation is, I use the term 'dynamic relaxation' to describe the type of relaxation being sought in this program, as opposed to the 'passive relaxation' that is involved with inactivity.

The FOF Program exercises recognise that the human body and mind are built around two basic response systems—the 'relaxation response' and the 'stress response' (sometimes called the 'flight or fight' response). To better understand what these responses are designed to achieve, it is perhaps better to think of them as the 'long-term survival response' and the 'short-term survival response'.

### THE 'RELAXATION' OR 'LONG-TERM SURVIVAL' RESPONSE

In this response, the body's energies and resources are focused on keeping the body healthy for as long as possible. This is the 'healing' mode, the state where the body's energies and resources are directed inwards for repair, maintenance and growth.

The energies of the body go towards such things as the immune system, which defends us against disease and infection, and the digestive system which nurtures and maintains us. It is the state where our organs and metabolic systems operate in a balanced and harmonious fashion that minimises long-term damage and strain on organs and tissues.

Tai Chi is one of the few exercise systems that is designed to operate with the body remaining in the relaxation response. Most other exercise systems, particularly those where the focus is on either competing against other people or various standards (composed of time, distance, height and so on), move the body into the stress response.

### THE 'STRESS' OR 'SHORT TERM SURVIVAL' RESPONSE

The stress response evolved to deal with life-threatening situations, even if this required operating in a mode that shortened one's total life expectancy. This is a reasonable trade-off. If a large bull is charging towards you then it makes sense that your body becomes much more concerned about surviving the next few seconds than it is about surviving the next few decades.

In the stress response, the body's resources are withdrawn from systems such as the immune and digestive systems and redirected outwards to muscular and energy-producing systems. Organs and metabolic processes are geared up to a level that ensures the body's short-term peak performance—no matter what the long-term damage done to organ and body systems. Blood is thickened and withdrawn from surface tissues and organs not essential to short-term survival so that not too much of this vital fluid is lost in the case of injury.

The stress response is like slamming on the brakes or flooring the accelerator when driving a car. It may get you out of an emergency situation but it dramatically increases the risk of mechanical failure and accident if used as a standard driving technique. Unfortunately, our bodies have not yet evolved to deal with today's modern environment and lifestyle, which continually create stimuli that puts the body into the stress response, even when the situations may not be life-threatening. In fact, the body's response to modern stresses is usually counterproductive.

Just think, when did getting stressed help you in an exam or an interview situation? Did being stressed improve how you handled that long traffic jam, the car breakdown, or the ATM eating your card? It's a lose–lose situation. There no real benefits to be gained, or even to balance the long-term damage being done, and the stress response usually makes things worse.

Does this mean that I am opposed to ever being stressed? Should we not compete in sports and business? Is having to meet a target or deadline bad for us? Not at all. The stress we feel when we abseil down a cliff, take a parachute jump or stand up in front of an audience to deliver a speech can provide an edge and focus that allows us to achieve more than we might otherwise. It can be stimulating and exhilarating.

There are also often-significant benefits derived from such exercises through the improvement of cardiovascular and other body functions. The danger is when such exercises simply serve as an aggravation of an already overstressed life and lead to the worsening of existing problems. The trick is to use the response correctly and to be able to relax quickly. For instance, if you're a rugby league player running towards the try line with half the other team thundering behind you, being in the stress response can be a real advantage that gives you an edge. Being in the stress response when you see a ball arcing towards you that you desperately want to catch can virtually guarantee a fumble as your hands and arms stiffen!

## Benefits of dynamic relaxation techniques

The techniques that achieve the relaxation response in physical exercise can be applied to many other activities in life including work, school and recreation. One of the great things about the FOF Program exercises is that, once their practice becomes a part of your regular routine, the techniques become second nature. They become unconsciously applied in many other areas of your life, helping to ensure that your body and mind remain as relaxed as possible throughout your day—not just while you practice the exercises.

There is a further stress-related benefit to be derived from dynamic relaxation techniques. This arises from the fact that the nature of the stimuli that cause stress responses in today's lifestyle and environment generally do not result in the release of stress. For example, we can guess that our average caveman became somewhat stressed when he found a sabre-tooth tiger close behind him. The 'flight or fight' that subsequently erupted would, if the caveman survived, release any built-up muscular tension and metabolise any adrenalin and other stress hormones that had been produced. Today, however, when we are caught in a traffic jam or queue, frustrated by the non-appearance of a meal we ordered, or suffering unfair criticism from our boss, there is no opportunity to release the built-up stress. This means that not only do we suffer stress during the stressful situation but for a long time after as well. These stored tensions have a number of deleterious effects, including a tendency to become more stressed (a vicious negative feedback cycle). The FOF Program exercises break this cycle by teaching us how to release these stored tensions.

# Appendix 2

# Healthy Posture

WE TEND TO THINK of posture as simply keeping a straight back to 'look good' but posture has an intimate relationship with not only how we look but also how we think and feel. It is about physical, mental and emotional balance. Further, posture affects our breathing, our digestion and our circulation of blood and lymph fluid. It is intimately tied up with our whole sense of being.

## A posture experiment

Posture affects mood dramatically. If you find this difficult to believe then try the following experiment:

- Stand with your feet shoulder width apart. Tilt your head forward, draw your shoulders slightly inwards and fix your eyes firmly on a spot on the floor between your feet.
- Without straightening up or raising your eyes, speak enthusiastically to a friend or family member about a recent enjoyable experience such as a holiday, a meal out, or a meeting with an old friend. Try

to recapture your mood and feeling and convey how much you enjoyed the experience. (If you can't think of an enjoyable experience then you definitely need Tai Chi!) How do you feel?

- Now straighten your spine, feeling as though your head is supported by a string connected to the crown of your head. Relax your whole body down from this point, look ahead, and deliver the same speech. Notice the difference in how you feel.

**CORRECT POSTURE POSITION**

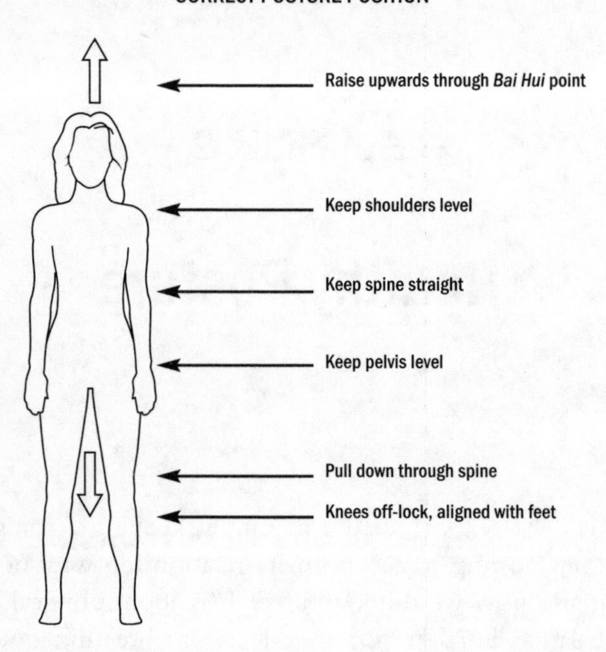


Posture affects the way you think and behave. Why else do you think the army spends so much time marching people about and standing them to attention? It helps to teach uncritical obedience. That might suggest something about the way that some schools teach! The process flows both ways, from body to mind and from mind to body—two sides of the same coin. Rigorous and uncompromising persons tend to reflect their attitude in their posture.

The FOF Program teaches you a relaxed upright posture that sits well with a feeling of mental expansiveness and optimism. From a Chinese perspective, the development of a relaxed and unconstricted flow of *Chi* throughout the body will be reflected in mental attitude. Also, there is a refined form of *Chi* known as *shen*. This can be translated as 'spirit'; though the French *élan vital* is a better description. (If you use the term spirit then it is used in the context of being 'high-spirited' or 'low-spirited'.) *Shen* has no religious significance, it is a Chinese medical term. In the West, when we ask a person how they feel, we are really asking 'What is the state of their *shen*?'

The FOF Program uses recognised techniques for raising the *shen*. When the *shen* is raised, the mood of depression disappears and an optimistic outgoing mood is encouraged. These techniques are borrowed from Tai Chi and are another reason why Tai Chi is regarded as an 'internal art'.

Appendix 3

# Healthy Movement Techniques

THE NATURE OF OUR MOVEMENT, like posture, is intimately related to our degree of relaxation and all the benefits that are attached to the relaxation response. The Chinese have long referred to a type of movement they call *Mian* or 'silk-like' movement. The name is derived both from the soft, flowing nature of silk, and from the traditional way of drawing the silken thread from the silkworm's cocoon—any jerkiness, any sudden changes in speed or direction and the delicate silk thread is broken. Your relaxation is as delicate as the silk thread. Move suddenly, move jerkily and it will be broken as you move into the stress response.

One useful piece of imagery for creating silk-like movement is to imagine that, when moving your hands, some very rare butterflies have landed on each of your hands and you do not want to disturb them before you can show somebody.

Transitions, from upwards to downwards, from left to right, from stillness to movement, from movement to stillness, are the areas to focus on. It is in transitions where abrupt movements and a break in the thread of your relaxation is likely to occur.

Appendix 4

# Healthy Breathing Techniques

HEALTHY BREATHING INVOLVES diaphragmatic breathing. This is where breathing is not forced but responsive, and the air is breathed into and out of the nose. As can be seen from the following, breathing and relaxation are linked in either mutually reinforcing or mutually destructive manner.

The prime objective of the breathing process is to maintain appropriate levels of oxygen and carbon dioxide within the blood. As metabolic activity increases (through exercise, for instance), oxygen is drawn out of the blood at a faster rate and the lungs must breathe in more air to replenish the oxygen that has been converted into the metabolic waste product of carbon dioxide.

It all sounds pretty simple but, in fact, the breathing or respiration process is amazingly subtle and sophisticated. Breathing is important not only to our continued existence, but also to our quality of life and state of vitality. So much so that it warrants our full understanding.

## Getting rid of some misconceptions

Perhaps the major misconception to get rid of is that if we need oxygen to live then the more oxygen we get the better. This is incorrect; too much oxygen in the blood is as bad as too little. Oxygen at higher levels than the body is programmed to maintain is a poison that can seriously damage the body!

The next misconception to get rid of is that if carbon dioxide is a waste product then we better get rid of as much of it as we can (usually by forced exhalation). Lowering carbon dioxide levels in our blood too far results in hyperventilation and interferes with a number of metabolic processes. The body has developed sophisticated chemical sensors that measure the chemical constitution of the blood, to ensure the appropriate level of oxygen and carbon dioxide is maintained. We breathe faster as we exercise because these sensors measure the rising proportion of carbon dioxide in the blood and trigger the inhalation process more frequently.

We should no more attempt to consciously interfere with the volume of air that these sensors determine is required in a given period of time than we should try to consciously interfere with the amount of blood that our heart is pumping. Unfortunately it is much easier to consciously interfere with our breathing than our heart rate. However, while our conscious brain can override the automatic breathing process, it has no way of determining what the oxygen needs of the body are, and will almost certainly cause us to breathe in too much or too little.

## Why do we need breathing exercises?

On the surface, it might sound as though we should not be doing breathing exercises at all, but the trick lies in understanding how to consciously influence the breathing pattern without changing the volume of air that the chemical sensors have determined is appropriate to breathe in over a given period of time.

There are still ways that we can influence the process because the volume of air we breathe in during a given time depends on two factors:

- the volume of air we inhale with each in-breath; and
- the number of breaths we take in each minute.

The existence of these two factors allows us to use our conscious mind and our automatic breathing processes together. For instance, if we consciously slow our breathing, the automatic breathing system responds by deepening the breath to make sure that the total volume of air breathed in over a given period of time remains at the appropriate level.

On the other hand, if we deepen our breathing then our automatic breathing system reduces the number of breaths we take per minute so that, again, the total volume of air remains appropriate.

This means that we can focus on either deepening our breath or slowing our breath so long as we do not try to do both at the same time. Does it make any difference to the body whether we take 12 breaths of one amount of air per minute or six breaths of twice that amount? The answer is a very definite 'yes' because the breathing function does not operate in isolation to other body systems.

Most of us know that when we are anxious, nervous or afraid we tend to breathe quickly and shallowly. This is an evolutionary device that shifts us into the stress response to prepare us for action. This made sense because when we lived in forests and jungles as it made the body be better prepared for 'fight or flight'. This is what the stress response is designed to prepare us for. The stress response, however, has a large number of negative impacts on long-term health including: shortening lifespan because of increased wear and tear on the body, and increased risk of disease and infection because of a run-down immune system.

Of course these negatives don't matter too much if the alternative is failing to survive the next few minutes! But, why breathe in a manner that causes these problems if there is no survival benefit?

Most of us know that when we are relaxed and at ease our breathing tends to be slow and deep. This was another evolutionary response. If the conscious mind was relaxed and at ease then there was probably no imminent threat and the body could concern itself with growth and maintenance. Of course, society has evolved faster than the body and now most of the threats we face in a modern world are better handled in a relaxed rather than stressed state. Think about driving, work relations, exams and so on. Do you do these better when you are stressed or relaxed? So in 'healthy breathing' we seek either to consciously slow our breath or consciously deepen our breath but never both!

## Techniques for consciously slowing the breath

There are three very simple techniques to consciously slow the breath:

- increasing the effective vital capacity of the lungs;
- breathing in and out through the nose; and
- having a mental awareness of the breath.

When we correct our posture and release tensions from the muscles, the effective vital capacity of our lungs increases because the lungs are not being compressed by postural and muscular distortion. When we breathe in and out through the nose, the nose simply cannot pass large volumes of air quickly so our breathing becomes slowed.

The simple act of becoming aware of the breath flowing into and out of the body slows down our breath rate. We are not consciously forcing the breath to be slower, we are simply becoming aware of the flow of air and how it feels as it passes through the nose, throat and lungs. We may become aware of the movements in the body torso, the rise and fall of the shoulders, the expansion and contraction of the abdomen, the wave-like motion that goes through the spine. Again, if we try to create these, we will only cause problems. It is the sense of listening with the senses that helps to slow your breathing.

Try this exercise: Focus on the feeling of the difference in the textures of the items of clothing that you are wearing at the moment. I would suspect that, while practicing this awareness exercise, you found that your breathing was slowing. This is not because you consciously tried to slow the movement but because you needed time to collect and evaluate the sensory data and your breathing automatically slowed to allow this to happen. The same process takes place in any breathing visualisation.

## Techniques for consciously deepening the breath

The depth of the breath (the volume of air taken into the lungs at each inhalation) can be adversely affected by a number of factors, including:

- tension in the shoulders (this reduces the amount by which the upper lungs can be expanded)'
- curvature of the spine (which compresses the internal organs and lungs together);
- abdominal tension (which reduces the movement of the lung diaphragm, thus reducing the amount by which the lower lungs can be expanded);
- stress or inactivity of the lung diaphragm (which again reduces lower-lung capacity).

All of the above factors cause reduction in the effective capacity of the lungs. This means that more breaths must be taken per minute to maintain required oxygen levels in the blood and the very fact of the faster breathing puts us back deeper into the stress response, establishing a negative feedback cycle that can be difficult to break.

There is another adverse impact of reduced lung capacity that should not be overlooked. The expansion and contraction of the lungs within the body torso create an internal massaging effect that assists in:

- Returning venous blood, which is depleted in oxygen and full of wastes and toxins, to the general circulatory system—this occurs when the lung diaphragm presses down on the internal organs, effectively squeezing out the venous blood.
- Supplying arterial blood, which is full of oxygen and nutrients, to the internal organs—this occurs when the lung diaphragm moves upwards, reducing the pressure in the abdominal cavity and causing internal organs to expand by drawing in fresh blood.
- Moving food through the intestinal tract, thus improving the digestive system.
- moving lymph fluid around the torso—lymph fluid is important in maintaining an effective immune system.

The FOF Program includes techniques and exercises for removal of tension in the shoulder area and for the correction of posture and spine. Techniques for removal of tension in the abdominal area and visualisation techniques also help to activate the lung diaphragm.

## Guidelines for healthy breathing during exercises

### BREATHE THROUGH THE NOSE

Unless we are performing an exertive activity (or have a severe cold), we should breathe in and out with the nose. From a physiological viewpoint, this process filters out airborne bacteria and helps to ensure that the air reaches the lungs at a temperature and humidity that is most appropriate for the health of the lungs.

When we undergo heavy exertion, we breathe in through the mouth. The reason for this is simple. When our metabolisms are operating at a high level, the amount of oxygen required to fuel the process goes up and we require a larger air intake more quickly, so we switch over to the mouth. In our evolution, this situation would have arisen when we were either obtaining food or seeking to avoid becoming food. In such situations the survival of the moment was most important. It makes sense to trade off some long-term health benefits to get through the next few life-threatening moments. Besides, if we are only breathing through the mouth for short periods of time, the negative health aspects are not likely to be particularly significant.

The important thing to remember is that nose breathing should be the method we use for more than 95 per cent of our breathing.

When you go to smell something, it is as though you focus the inward breath on the inner tip of the nose. This would have been an important survival characteristic in the past when the scent of danger or food was something that we needed to know about as soon as possible. These things are so unimportant today that we rarely use this skill.

This is a pity because there is an acupoint at the tip of the nose called *Su Liao* and this point becomes activated when we draw in air to the tip of the nose. This is the first point at which a linkage between the body's energetic systems and the *Chi* in the air becomes established. When you consider the important relationship between certain aromas and our body's overall state, such as lavender and relaxation, the implications of the disuse of this acupoint is something that warrants more study than it has received up to now.

Finally, do not snort or sniff. The air should be taken into the nose smoothly and quietly. The key is mentally focusing on the tip of the nose. The benefits of breathing through the nose include:

- encourages relaxation;
- protects lungs against infection and allergens;
- protects lungs against temperature and moisture stress;
- encourages the use of the lung diaphragm;
- increased calmness with initiation of the body's relaxation response and reduction of stress and anxiety levels;
- increased feeling of vitality and well-being;
- improves operation of the immune system;
- increases internal massaging effects of the lung diaphragm on the internal organs, thus improving the supply of arterial blood and the removal of venous blood;
- opens of the capillary network, improving blood supply to the cells.

### PLACE THE TONGUE AGAINST THE ROOF OF THE MOUTH

Breathing through the nose has the additional benefit of it being possible to keep the tip of the tongue against the roof of the mouth while breathing. This forms a physical connection between the end of the *Du Mai* meridian and the starting point of the *Ren Mai* meridian, completing the Microcosmic Orbit and greatly encouraging the flow of energy therein. This position also increases the production of saliva, which aids digestion and increases the immune system's defences in the mouth.

### USE THE LUNG DIAPHRAGM

Diaphragmatic breathing has, as well as all its useful physiological benefits, a stimulatory effect on the energetic centre known as the *Tan Tien*. The inward movement of the abdomen with the out-breath and the outward movement with the in-breath are good indications of the proper movement the lung diaphragm.

Unfortunately the lung diaphragm is particularly susceptible to stress and tension and it may take some time to relax this area and get the diaphragm to do its job. The benefits are well worthwhile and include:

- greatly increased lung capacity;
- internal massaging effects on the internal organs that improve their blood circulation—resulting in them receiving nutrients and removing waste products more efficiently—and the health and functioning of the internal organs, which is vital to overall health;
- internal massaging effects on the large and small intestines, assisting the peristaltic process and improving the efficiency of digestion;
- internal massaging effects on the lymphatic system—this is a key part of our immunological defence system and its circulation relies on massaging effects provided primarily by lungs and muscles.

### USE VISUALISATION, NOT MENTAL CONTROL

Even though the air finishes it's journey in the lungs, it is helpful to picture the breath flowing downwards to the *Chi Hai* point. The visualised stream of air should be mentally followed from the nose, down the throat, and then just under the skin, from the base of the throat, along the centreline of the body. In other words, the path along which the air flows is the same as the trajectory of the *Ren Mai* meridian, and the direction of flow of breath and flow of *Chi* are in the same direction.

With the exhalation, the air is returned from the lungs to the nose. To visualise the flow of air, imagine the air moving up the centre of the back, just under the skin, to the base of the neck. Then follow the sensation of the air up the throat and out of the nose. In other words, the upward, outward path of the air follows the *Du Mai* meridian.

A more advanced version of this breathing technique can be performed by initially directing the outward breath of the air downwards to the *Hui Yin* acupoint on the perineum then upward along the spine to the crown of the head at the *Bai Hui* acupoint and downwards again to the *Su Liao* point. Effectively, this breathing opens up the entire Microcosmic Circulation but this is a very powerful breathing technique that may have some side effects if not approached in a controlled manner and with considerable knowledge of the Microcosmic Orbit. Certainly, if you are attempting this breathing pattern and you feel any physical or mental discomfort, focus the mind back to the *Tan Tien* and centre your energy there.

The most important acupoint involved in breathing is the *Chi Hai* acupoint—its name means 'sea of *Chi*'. This acupoint is found about three finger widths below the navel, and while the *Chi Hai* point lies on the *Du Mai* meridian, it is also the connection point with the *Tan Tien*. Mentally focusing on the *Chi Hai* acupoint greatly increases the *Chi* that is absorbed from breathing.

### IMPORTANT WARNING ABOUT HEALTHY BREATHING

Healthy breathing is mainly about the mental focus that we apply when breathing as well as some physiological aspects, such as breathing through the nose and using diaphragmatic breathing. It does not require forcing the breath or mentally overriding the depth and frequency of your breathing. Doing this can cause discomfort and can even be dangerous. Develop the art of listening (with your ears and your body) to your breath. Your breathing will change naturally as you become aware of what you are doing. There is no need to control it.

Taking too much air into the lungs too rapidly floods your body with oxygen. This is called hyperventilation and has all sorts of negative effects. On the other extreme, breathing too shallowly or too infrequently is called hypoventilation and this can deprive the brain of the required oxygen, resulting in fainting. If you have any breathing condition, the exercises detailed in this book should assist your health but seek your doctor's advice first.

Appendix 5

# The Energy System

TO UNDERSTAND HOW the *Chi* energy system works within the human body, it is necessary to become familiar with a number of terms:

## The meridians

Each person's body has its own *Chi* field, although the basic structure of this field is the same for everyone. To be consistent with the majority of literature on the subject, we will refer to the 'lines of force' or 'energy trajectories' within these *Chi* fields as meridians. The meridians in the body are divided up into two major groups: organ meridians and extraordinary meridians.

| | |
|---|---|
| Organ meridians | These are associated with the health and functioning of specific organ systems. There are 12 organ meridians: heart, lungs, spleen, liver, kidneys, pericardium, small intestine, large intestine, stomach, gall bladder, bladder, and triple heater. |

| | |
|---|---|
| Extraordinary meridians | These are associated with the balancing and distribution of *Chi* energy throughout the body. There are eight extraordinary meridians: *Du Mai* (Governing Vessel), *Ren Mai* (Conception Vessel), *Chong Mai* (Ocean Vessel), *Dai Mai* (Belt Vessel), *Yang Chiao Mai*, *Yin Chiao Mai*, *Yang Wei Mai*, and *Yin Wei Mai*. |

*Chi* flows along the meridians, flowing in the organ meridians in a specific direction. It is better to visualise this flow like water or blood, as *Chi* flows relatively slowly. This does not contradict its energy nature. Changes in magnetic fields can also be relatively slow.

### HOW CAN THE FLOW OF *CHI* THROUGH A MERIDIAN BE CHANGED?

There are a number of ways the flow of *Chi* through a meridian can be influenced. They include:

- Mental concentration on the flow of *Chi*, either by the individual or by a trained *Chi* practitioner. The focus can be either on moving an imaginary ball of *Chi* along the pathway of the meridian, or in sequence, on the major acupoints in the meridian. Both these techniques are *Chi* meditation techniques.
- Brushing the hands lightly along the pathway of the meridian while focusing on energy movement in the meridian. This is called 'meridian brushing'.
- Performing specific movements and exercises. In a sense, *Chi* can be compared to water in a pipe or channel—if the pipe or channel is straight, the water flows faster; when the pipe or channel is bent or curved, the flow is slower.
- Performing exercises that straighten the *Chi* meridians, stimulating a faster flow of energy. It should also be remembered that this is a system of interconnected channels and, by properly planned movements, one can shift *Chi* from one channel to another.
- Chinese massage techniques for muscles and joints will increase the flow of *Chi* in the meridians where it passes through the area being massaged. Importantly, the person receiving the massage should be comfortable both physically and mentally. Any stress or tension

caused by over-zealous philosophy of 'no pain, no gain' may actually cause a reduction in the amount of *Chi* that is flowing.
- *Chi* flow through the meridians may also be increased by stimulating the acupoints lying on the meridians—for example, by acupuncture, acupressure, moxabustion or stimulation with a laser or electrical current, or any combination thereof.

Each meridian is associated with a particular frequency of vibration and colour, thus the visualisation of colour can stimulate energy flows in particular organ meridians. There are herbs that have specific effects on *Chi* flow, with certain sounds and scents also having a specific impact.

**THE DIFFERENCES BETWEEN THE ORGAN AND EXTRAORDINARY MERIDIANS:**
- Extraordinary meridians have no acupoints unique to themselves, rather they share points on various organ meridians and can thus move energy between different meridians.
- Extraordinary meridians are not related to any particular organ.
- Extraordinary meridians do not flow in one particular direction. Rather, they flow from the area of highest concentration of *Chi* to the area of lowest concentration. If there is no differential in energy levels between two points, then there is no flow of energy.
- Extraordinary meridians are regarded as being more responsive to mental states than organ meridians.

Two of the extraordinary meridians contradict the above rules: the *Du Mai* and *Ren Mai* share the characteristics of both extraordinary and organ meridians in that:

- they are respectively associated with the brain and reproductive organs;
- they have their own acupoints;
- whilst the energy can flow different ways in the meridians, one particular way is regarded as more usual;
- they are concerned with balancing energy in other meridians.

Because their energy-balancing functions are so important, the *Du Mai* and *Ren Mai* are generally classed with the extraordinary meridians. While there has been much focus on the organ meridians in the West, the extraordinary meridians should also be seen as critical to the maintenance of health.

### THE EXTRAORDINARY MERIDIANS

The extraordinary meridians divide into three important sub-categories:

- Microcosmic Circulation
- Macrocosmic Circulation
- Additional Extraordinary Meridians

#### Microcosmic Circulation

This is the name given to the energy circuit formed by the *Du Mai* and *Ren Mai*. These two meridians form the prime energy circuit on which the rest of the energy system depends. If the flow of *Chi* within the Microcosmic Circuit is not healthy, then problems will develop elsewhere. The Microcosmic Circuit must always be the first point of focus in the meridians. To use an analogy, this circuit is like the main line of a railway system. It would be asking for trouble to develop traffic on the branch lines if the main line was already handling its limit.

As previously noted, the *Du Mai* and *Ren Mai* also serve as the organ meridians for the brain and reproductive organs, which is reflected in their names, originally translated as Governing Vessel and Conception Vessel.

#### Macrocosmic circulation:

This, as the name would imply, is an extension of the microcosmic circuit. It includes six extraordinary meridians. This circuit of energy should be the next point of focus after the Microcosmic Circuit.

The *Yin Wei M* and *Yang Wei M* are known as the Great Regulator channels. The *Yin Wei Mo* connects with all the *Yin* meridians—spleen, liver, lung, pericardium, kidney and heart. The *Yang Wei Mo* connects with all the *Yang* meridians—stomach, gall bladder, bladder, large intestine, small intestine and triple heater. The *Yin Chiao Mo* and *Yang Chiao Mo* are known as the Great Bridge Channels; their function is to balance the energy of the *Yin* meridians with that of the *Yang* meridians.

#### Additional extraordinary meridians:

These additional extraordinary meridians are of great significance. In Taoist philosophy, the *Chong Mai* is listed with the *Du Mai* and *Ren Mai* and these are known as the three great psychic channels. The *Chong Mai* (or Penetrating Vessel) runs from the mouth, down through/over the lungs, through the general area of the *Tan Tien* to *Hui Yin*; branches go down the legs, up through the kidneys, and along the inside of the spine. In fact, in many ways, the abdominal *Tan Tien* may be regarded as part of the *Chong Mai* and perhaps, for this reason, the Taoists attribute to *Chong Mai* the capacity to store *Chi* energy. There is considerable disputation in classical texts about the exact configuration of *Chong Mai*.

The last extraordinary meridian is the *Dai Mai*, or Belt Meridian, which, apart from its general energy regulation effect, is also believed to be associated with the protection of energy in the *Tan Tien*.

### GENERAL OBSERVATIONS ON THE PATHWAYS OF MERIDIANS

It must be appreciated that the meridians thread and weave their way through the human body, sometimes rising to the surface, at other times penetrating to the core. Only those portions of the meridians on the surface have accessible acupoints. Often, for the sake of simplicity and because the focus is on intervening with the existing flow of *Chi*, many books show only the accessible parts of meridian pathways. This can present a distorted view of the nature and function of the meridians.

The branches of the meridians that lie on the surface of the body are actually the least important aspect of the meridian. It is the internal part of the meridian, moving deep in the body tissue and closely associated with the internal organs, that is its vital part.

This helps to clear up the confusion of how the *Tan Tien* connects with the meridian system. When one explores the internal pathways of the meridians, one finds that they all pass through the area known as *Tan Tien*, which is situated just in front of the descending aorta and ascending venae cavae, immediately between the two kidneys. This area was known to the ancient Chinese as the area of 'moving' *Chi*. (Since *jieng* is stored in the kidneys, it also provides the linking point between *jieng* and *Chi*.)

Basically, when the amount of *Chi* energy falls below the required amount, *jieng* is converted into *Chi* which is then available to flow through the meridian system. Whether this conversion mechanism can reverse is the subject of much speculation and disagreement. It therefore seems wise to err on the side of caution and thus avoid situations which tend to activate the *jieng* conversion process.

The inner trajectories of the meridians were fully specified in *The*

*Yellow Emperor's Classic of Internal Medicine*. Modern practitioners still find these observations valid.

Whilst, to date, there has been no conclusive identification of the bodily structures which carry *Chi*, there is a growing belief that this is, or relates to, the fascial tissue within the body. Bio-electric currents have been measured travelling along this tissue and there is nothing within the structure of the fascial tissue that contradicts the energy trajectories identified by the Chinese. Since we know this tissue has connections, not only between cells but within them, it provides a communication network within the body of the same order, or greater, than the nervous system.

## The acupoints

Acupoints are specific locations on the surface of the body which have been identified as both reflecting the internal state of *Chi* and, through various treatment methods, being able to correct and bring the body's *Chi* into balance. Almost a thousand such points have been identified, although knowledge of only 20 or 30 acupoints is quite adequate for many basic *Chi* management techniques.

Most of the acupoints lie on the organ meridians. There are also some points on two of the extraordinary meridians—the *Du Mai* and *Ren Mai*. As well as these, there are a small number of acupoints with no known relation to any meridian. The most well-known of these would probably be *Yin Tang* (immediately between the eyebrows).

Whilst the term 'acupoint' is in common use in the West, it is misleading for a number of reasons.

Firstly, the term 'acu' means 'needle' (and obviously has been inherited from accupuncturists). This suggests that the point is simply something to be needled. In actual fact, acupoints can be used for diagnosis as well as for treatment, with the sensitivity and feel of the acupoint revealing much about the underlying condition of *Chi*.

Secondly, there are many other applicable treatment modes (in fact, needling should be the last resort). Points can be stimulated by thought, massage, negative and positive pressure, heat and moxa, electro-stimulation and laser, and by the application of magnets.

Thirdly, the word 'point' implies something minute and precisely located. Following the location description of an acupoint, however, is only a start. Acupoints move within the local area, thus it must be sensed or felt and not simply assumed to be in a particular location.

The original Chinese expression for acupoint was *Hsueh*, meaning 'hole', 'cavity' or 'cave'. This gives a much better sense of the acupoint as something lying hidden under the surface, which can be empty or full and which must be sought out.

### ACUPOINT RELEASE, TONING AND SEDATION

The first thing to establish with any acupoint is that the *Chi* energy can flow freely. Often, because of stress and tension within the body, the free flow of *Chi* energy is blocked. Therefore, standard techniques aim to release or open up the point. Basically, opening a point is done by loosening the tissue around the point. The use of one's own *Chi* energy can help to break through a blockage. Remembering that the *Chi* energy on organ meridians has one direction of flow, one should always work with this flow when working on any organ meridian acupoint. (No damage is done if one works opposite to the flow but neither is there any benefit.)

With the exception of the *Du Mai* and *Ren Mai*, extraordinary meridians always flow in the direction of lowest energy. Extraordinary meridians have no unique acupoints and therefore can be disregarded for basic acupressure work.

The *Du Mai* and *Ren Mai* meridians do have unique acupoints and their direction of *Chi* energy flow can vary. In general terms, working with the direction of energy flow tones or stimulates the energy while working against the direction of energy flow sedates or calms the energy.

### MENTAL STIMULATION OF ACUPOINTS

The fact that the mind can be used to change the flow of energy at acupoints should not be surprising. Focus of attention on one point of the body often increases sensitivity (have you ever watched a mosquito bite you and distinctly felt the process of the normally undetectable bite?) and causes other physiological changes. Most people can increase blood flow and raise the temperature by at least 1°C in any point of the body on which they choose to focus.

### *TAN TIEN*

There are three *Tan Tien* in the human body—the upper, middle, and lower. If not otherwise designated, it is the lower *Tan Tien* that is usually being referred to. This is the *Tan Tien* which most concerns us during exercise breathing and Qigong.

What constitutes a *Tan Tien* is very difficult to explain. They are not meridians or acupoints, rather they are areas associated with particular refinements of *Chi* energy. (Interestingly, the location of the three *Tan Tien* is in accordance with three of the chakras, as in yoga.)

**Lower *Tan Tien*:**

This is the area which equates to the *Hara*, located about three finger widths below the navel in the centre of the torso. *Tan* means 'pill', or 'immortality'; *Tien* means 'field'. The *Chi Hai* acupoint is immediately in front of the *Tan Tien*; the *Ming Men* to the rear.

*The Yellow Emperor's Classic of Internal Medicine* states that the, 'moving *Chi* between the kidneys' is the source of all the body's *Chi*. What does this mean? Post-birth *Chi* is obtained from air, food and environment; pre-natal *Chi* is stored within the kidneys. Perhaps the expression 'root of the body's *Chi*' describes the image better.

The lower *Tan Tien* is seen as important because this is where the *Chi* is 'stored'. However, the extraordinary meridians are also known to play a role in *Chi* storage. The essential role of *Tan Tien* might be found in the fact that this is the store of energy which determines whether or not we draw on *jieng* and thus deplete our potential lifespan.

To understand the relationship between the organ meridians and the *Tan Tien*, imagine a set of battery-powered Christmas tree lights, able to operate off mains power when it is available but switch over to battery power when it is not. Each organ is represented by a different light; the wire that leads into each light is the organ meridian; the mains power/battery is the *Tan Tien*.

Anybody who has put up Christmas-tree lights knows that, because the electrical circuit leads from wire to light to next wire to next light and so on, one loose connection and the whole circuit fails to work. Such a system failure would be catastrophic in a living system and there needs to be redundancy in the system to help it to overcome system faults that might develop. This is, in essence, the role of the extraordinary meridians, which act like cross-connected wires, able to take the power around faults in the system and keep the whole process going.

This explanation is, of course, simplistic. The human *Chi* system is a lot more complicated and sophisticated, having much more in common with a national power grid and the way in which it is operated—to keep power flowing to meet complex sets of demands—than it does with a set of Christmas-tree lights. However, the basic principle is the same.

**Middle *Tan Tien*:**
In males, the middle *Tan Tien* is located behind the sternum, at the same height as the nipples; in females, it is located about an inch and a half from the base of the sternum, technically on a level with the fourth intercostal space.

**Upper *Tan Tien*:**
This is located at the same height as the eyebrows, directly behind the centre point between them.

# Glossary

**Acumassage:** The use of physical pressure and manipulation on the acupoints to correct flows of *Chi* energy.

**Acupressure:** *see* Acumassage.

**Acupuncture:** The use of needles to penetrate and stimulate acupoints to correct the flows of *Chi* energy.

**Allergy:** An over-sensitisation of the immune system to organic and inorganic chemicals.

**Assimilation:** The absorption of nutrients from the intestines into the bloodstream.

***Bai Hui*:** An important acupoint for vitality and energy. It is found at the crown of the head

**Bio feedback:** The return of an output, such as heart rate, blood pressure etc, as an input or stimulus, with the objective of modifying the output.

**Chan San Feng:** The legendary creator of Tai Chi.

***Chi:*** The name given to the vital energy that drives all activity in the universe.

***Chi* breathing:** Breathing techniques that focus on the extraction of *Chi* from the air.

***Chi* diet:** A form of diet where the focus is on the quantity, nature and quality of the *Chi* that is obtained from food.

***Chi* Kung:** Literally, 'skill with energy'.

***Chi* meditation:** The use of mental focus to encourage the proper flow of *Chi* throughout the body.

**Chen-style Tai Chi:** The first historical form of Tai Chi. It is a fairly vigorous martial art.

***Chi Hai*:** An important acupoint that is three finger widths below the navel. It enables the extraction of *Chi* from the breathing process.

**Colon:** Another name for the large intestine. It functions are the retention of water and the elimination of waste product.

**Conception Vessel:** *see Ren Mai* meridian.

***Dao Yin*:** A Chinese exercise system, developed more than 2500 years ago, that focused on breathing, posture and energy circulation. It is sometimes called *Tao Yin*.

**Diaphragmatic breathing:** Breathing that is primarily driven by the lung diaphragm, moving downwards on the in-breath and moving upwards on the out-breath

**Digestion:** The process of breaking down complex nutrients into simpler nutrients. It takes place in the digestive tract.

***Du Mai:*** Also called the Governing Vessel, it is a meridian that runs up the centre of the back, over the head, and down the centre front of the head.

**Endocrine glands:** Glands that secrete hormones that modify metabolic and growth activity within the body.

**Five elements theory:** The theory that deals with the five elemental energy phases of *Chi*—wood, fire, earth, metal and water.

**Extraordinary meridians:** The name given to the eight meridians that deal with the balancing of energy within the body.

**Genetic predisposition:** The increased likelihood of developing a particular condition because of one's genetic heritage

**Governing Vessel:** *see Du Mai* meridian.

***Hegu:*** An important acupoint for vitality and energy. It is found in the fleshy tissue between the thumb and index finger.

**Horse-riding stance:** An important exercising stance with straight back, bent knees and the sensation of gripping a horse with the legs.

***Hsueh:*** The Chinese name for acupoint which more correctly describes the area as a cavern of *Chi*.

**Immune function/system:** The body's systems that deal with defence against infection and injury.

**Intercostal muscles:** The muscles that expand the upper rib cage and are used in chest breathing.

***Lao Gong*:** An important acupoint at the centre of the palm.

**Large intestine:** *see* Colon.

**Large intestine meridian:** The energy meridian that is paired with the lung meridian.

**Lotus body-toning relaxation system**: *Chi Kung* exercise system used in AATC.

**Lung capacity vital:** The total volume of air that the lungs can take in on a single breath.

**Lung capacity effective:** The total volume of air that is actually taken in on a single breath due to postural and muscular problems; always less than the vital capacity.

**Lung diaphragm:** The sheet of muscle that separates the chest and abdominal cavity and is used in diaphragmatic breathing.

**Lymph:** The fluid that is circulated through the body and lymphatic system which has much to do with the control of infection.

**Lymphatic system:** The system that generates and filters the lymph fluid.

**Medical advisor:** The primary health consultant, for example, a registered medical practitioner or other health consultant if you have chosen a practitioner from the alternative health care area.

***Meng Mun:*** A very important acupoint on the spine opposite the navel.

**Meridian:** An energy channel that carries *Chi*.

***Mian:*** Silk-like movement, that is, movement without jerkiness or abrupt changes of direction.

**Microcosmic Circulation:** The energy circulation pathway that is formed by the *Du Mai* and *Ren Mai* meridians.

**Moxabustion:** The burning of moxa herbs over acupoints to stimulate energy flow.

**Nasal breathing:** In-breath and out-breath through the nose.

***Nei Guan:*** An acupoint about three finger widths from the crease of the wrist in the centre of the underside of the arm, between the tendons.

**Off-lock position:** The release of the full extension or "lock" of a joint. It creates a slight bend of the joint to allow the muscles to absorb any shocks that could harm the joints.

**Organ meridian:** An energy channel that supports an organ function.

**Osteoporosis:** The loss of calcium from bones that results in increased risk of breakage and fracture.

**Oxygen debt**: The drop of oxygen levels in the blood due to sudden vigorous exercise.

**Peristalsis:** The wave-like motion that passes through the muscles of the wall of the intestines or oesophagus to assist the passage of food or fluids.

**Positive thinking:** Various mental techniques that use positive imagery and affirmation within thought.

**Reflexology:** The recognition that the body has a holistic nature and that various parts of the body have relationships to other parts (often far removed). Massage or manipulation of these 'reflex zones' or 'reflex points' can be used to influence the functioning of the connected point.

***Ren Mai:*** Also called the Conception Vessel, this extraordinary meridian runs down the front centre of the body torso.

**Respiratory system:** The system that deals with the taking in of oxygen and the release of carbon dioxide from the body.

***Shen:*** The spirit in the sense of being in a high-spirited, state of the emotional energy and feeling of well-being.

**Shibashi:** A series of 18 Tai Chi *Chi Kung* exercises, popular in China and taught by the AATC as an introductory Tai Chi *Chi Kung.*

**Silk-like movement:** *see Mian*

***Su Liao* point:** An acupoint at tip of nose that is involved in breathing.

**Tai Chi:** An abbreviation for Tai Chi Chuan, which means "the supreme ultimate fist". It also describes any exercise that contains the principles outlined in the Tai Chi Ching, involving relaxation, breathing, posture, slow movement, *Mian, Chi Kung* techniques, and martial-arts applications.

**Tai Chi breathing:** Breathing that involves unforced diaphragmatic breathing with inhalation and exhalation through the nose.

**Tai Chi Ching:** The classic writings on Tai Chi by masters such as Chan San Feng.

**Tai Chi massage:** Massage techniques that focus on relaxation, the flow of *Chi*, and posture.

**Tai Chi stretching:** Involves the use of muscles against each other rather than against the joints. There is never a full extension of the limbs, rather one extends the limb and simultaneously pulls it back.

***Tao*:** This literally means 'the way' that the universe operates and evolves. It is sometimes called the *Dao*.

***Tao Yin:*** *see Dao Yin.*

**Taoist:** A follower of the *Tao*.

***Tan Tien:*** The area in front of and between the kidneys, where the body stores *Chi*.

**Tiger's Mouth:** The inside edge of the first finger and thumb which form a mouth-like shape.

**Venous blood return system:** The system of veins, venous valves and muscles that acts to pump the blood back towards the heart as the limbs are moved during physical activity.

***Wei Chi:*** The defensive energy enveloping the body preventing infection. In Chinese terms, bacteria and viruses infect the body when *Wei Chi* is weak.

***Wai Guan:*** The acupoint (Triple Heater 8) about three finger widths from the crease of the wrist in the centre of the upper side of the forearm.

***Yang:*** The positive active nature of *Chi*.

**Yang-style Tai Chi:** The Tai Chi form devised by the Yang family.

***Yin:*** The passive, gathering nature of *Chi*.

***Yin–Yang* theory:** The theory that *Chi* has two basic natures, *Yin* and *Yang*, that need to be balanced and harmonised.

***Yun Men:*** The chief lung meridian acupoint.

# Resources

Further resources are available from the AATC to supplement and develop the material provided in this book. The AATC is happy to assist and can be contacted at:

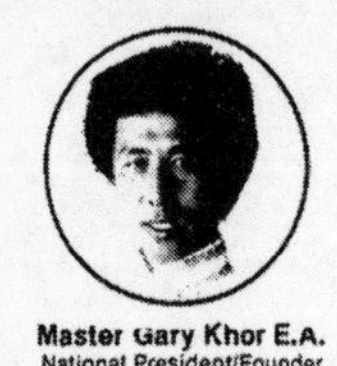


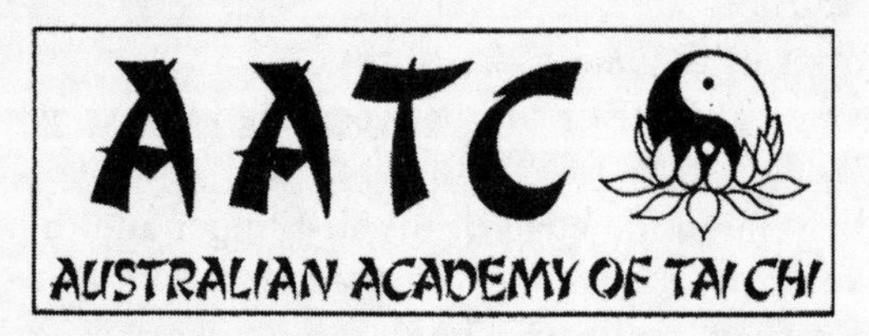


**Website: www.livingchi.com.au**
**email: aatch@optushome.com.au**

STATE OFFICES

**New South Wales**
(National Head Office)
686 Parramatta Road
Croydon NSW 2132
(PO Box 1020,
Burwood North NSW 2134)
Tel: (02) 9797 9355

**South Australia**
GPO Box 1306
Adelaide SA 5001
Tel: (08) 8287 3571

**Queensland**
PO Box 2475
Fortitude Valley BC Qld 4006
Tel: (07) 3358 1955

**Tasmania**
PO Box 1688
Launceston TAS 7250
Tel: 0438 346 620

**Western Australia**
7 Crofton Place
Lynwood WA 7147
Tel: (08) 9258 3434
email: westchi@iprimus.com.au

### REGIONAL OFFICES

**New South Wales**
Albury (02) 6043 2982
Ballina (02) 6686 5853
Baradine (02) 6843 1982
Bundanoon (02) 4883 6077
Central Coast (02) 4332 7176
Coonabarabran (02) 6482 2079
Corowra (02) 6033 3172
Deniliquin (03) 5881 5707
Kootingal (02) 6765 8292
Newcastle (02) 4942 2951
Orange (02) 6365 8309
Tamworth (02) 6765 8292
Wagga Wagga (02) 6931 7351
Woolongong (02) 4261 5786

**Queensland**
Bundaberg (07) 4153 7739
Gold Coast (07) 5572 8921
Rockhampton (07) 4928 6562
Sunshine Coast (07) 5491 2314
Toowoomba (07) 4636 5034

### EDUCATIONAL SERVICES

**Standard courses:** Community courses are held in most areas. Private instruction is also available.
**Seminars and workshops:** These are held regularly in main centres. Grandmaster Khor and others are also available to visit your area and present a workshop or seminar. Corporate, children's and seniors' packages, talks and demonstrations, including guest speakers, can be tailored to your needs.
Instruction training courses and business franchises are available.

## HOME LEARNING AND COURSE BACK-UP

**Videos:**

*Tai Chi for Health and Relaxation*
*Stress Control the Eastern Way*
*Qigong Shibashi: The 18 Techniques*
*Khor Tai Chi: Moving Meditation*
*Wellness Exercise: Lotus, Lohan and Sword*

**Music Tapes:**

Exclusive oriental music for Tai Chi and Qigong exercises is available. Also available are tapes excellent for meditation, relaxation, background music or just easy listening.

'Beginnings'—peaceful and relaxing
'Tao Yin'—oriental bamboo flute and string music
'Lohan'—beautiful Qigong music
'Tai Chi'—music for relaxation

# Bibliography

Jingfeng, Cai, *Eating Your Way to Health—Dietotheraphy in traditional Chinese medicine*, Foreign Language Press (China), 1988.

Khor, Gary, *Feng Shui for Personal Harmony*, Simon & Schuster (Australia), 2000.

— *Living Chi*, Simon & Schuster (Australia), 2001.

— *Tai Chi for a Healthy Lifestyle*, New Holland Publishers (Australia), 2000.

— *Tai Chi for Better Breathing*, Simon & Schuster (Australia), 2001.

— *Tai Chi for Stress Control*, Simon & Schuster (Australia), 1990.

Lane, Donald J., *Asthma; The Facts*, Oxford University Press, 1996.

Meek, Jennifer, and Holford, Patrick, *Boost Your Immune System*, Judy Piatkus (Publishers) Ltd.

Pearsall, Paul, PhD, *The Hearts Code*, Batam Book, 1999.

Robinson, Jo, and Barrett, Kathy, *Caring For Your Feet*, Choice Book 2000.

Schneider, Meir, and Larkin, Maureen, *The Handbook Of Self Healing,* Aekana Penquin Books, 1994.

— and Larkin, Maureen, *The Handbook Of Self Healing*, Aekana Penquin Books, 1994.

Sobel, Dava, and Klien, Arthur C., *Arthritis*, The Book Company, 1998.

St Vincents Hospital, the Diabetes Centre, *Understanding Diabetes*, Simon & Schuster, 1997.

Thompson, Sue, and Kelly, Dr Paul, *Healthy Bones*, Hodder & Stoughton, 1997.

Veith, Inza, *The Yellow Emperor's Classic of Internal Medicine*, University of California Press, 1972.

# Index